MW00526994

Healing Chronic Illness
By His Spirit, Through His Resources

"With candor, clarity, and compassion, Connie Strasheim hits two of the fuzziest subjects that I know of head-on: mystery illnesses and faith healing. She slices into the vagaries of both of these discussions with refreshing matter-of-factness, as she skillfully dissects the conventional wisdom, and offers balanced, practical guidance for the chronically ill. Deeply informative and filled with sincere faith, her insights will give hope to many who desperately need it."

— Rob Brendle
Senior Pastor
Denver United Church
www.denverunited.com
Author of *In The Meantime: The Practice of Proactive Waiting*

"I have known Connie for many years and she is a top notch researcher and writer. Having said this, you might be amazed that she is an even better person. Her integrity is unmatched, and her resolve is unwavering. As I helped her proofread this book, I sensed something special going on, not just in the book, but all over Colorado. A rising tide of change is coming upon us; healing, restoration, encouragement and life. Many books sit on the shelves for years, just waiting to be tasted. Don't miss this one—move it to the top of the pile and be blessed. It only takes a little faith, a little action and a little belief to see God move. Take that step today and watch everything change for the better."

— Rick Roberts
President, Legacy Grace Ministry
Author, dreamer, father, teacher

Also by Connie Strasheim:

Insights Into Lyme Disease Treatment:
13 Lyme-Literate Health Care Practitioners Share Their
Healing Strategies
(also available in Spanish)

The Lyme Disease Survival Guide:
Physical, Lifestyle, and Emotional Strategies
For Healing

Available for purchase from the author at
www.LymeBytes.blogspot.com

Or from the publisher at
www.LymeBook.com

Healing Chronic Illness
By His Spirit, Through His Resources

By **Connie Strasheim**

BioMed Publishing Group
P.O. Box 550531
South Lake Tahoe, CA 96155

To order additional copies of this book, visit www.healingchronicillness.org

Disclaimer

This book is not intended as medical advice. It is also not intended to prevent, diagnose, treat or cure disease. Instead, the book is intended only to share the author's opinion on the topic of spiritual healing, as would an investigative journalist. The book is provided for informational and educational purposes only, not as treatment instructions for any disease. Much of the book is a statement of opinion in areas where the facts are controversial or do not exist.

If you have a medical problem, please consult a licensed physician; this book is not a substitute for professional medical care. The statements in this book have not been evaluated by the FDA.

Acknowledgements

I want to say thank you to all those who, indirectly or directly, influenced the writing of this book.

To Rick Roberts and Karla Johnson, my spiritual mentors, for your valuable input on the book's content.

To Kristin Zhivago, who has helped me through the trials of chronic illness, encouraged me in my writing, and given me sound advice in all of my spiritual and business endeavors.

To my parents, John and Karen, for providing for me when I was too sick to provide for myself.

To my friends in the Lyme disease community, for sharing your stories with me, and for allowing me to share mine with you. Your lives have inspired me to write this book.

To the ministers who influenced my theology on healing, especially Bill Johnson: thank you for shining the light of God's truth upon my spirit and soul. Since I learned of your teachings, I have walked in unprecedented freedom in the Spirit.

To Bryan Rosner, my publisher, for going above and beyond to get this book published in a timely manner, and for believing in me as a writer of not only medical books, but also spiritual healing books.

And finally, to Jesus Christ, my healer and redeemer. It is because of You that I can experience Heaven on earth, as well as in the afterlife. To You be all the glory, honor and praise...forever and ever. Amen.

Table of Contents

Foreword   11

Chapter 1
God's Will for Our Wellness and What Led Me to Believe   **13**

The God of Love, the God of Miracles   14
My Story and the Stepping Stones of Faith   16
God's Plan for Our Lives   24

Chapter 2
Why God May Allow Disease   **27**

Our Faith Is in Medicine   28
By Our Trials We Are Ultimately Made Well   29
Sickness Forces Us to Face Our Demons   30
Sickness Teaches Us How to Develop Healthy Habits   31
Sickness Teaches Us Dependence upon Him   33
Sickness Motivates Us to Change Our Thoughts   35
Only Those Who Have "Been There, Suffered That" Are Qualified to Empathize with the Sick   37
Disease Motivates Us to Advance Our Knowledge of Medicine to Heal Others   39
Disease Teaches Us to Set Healthy Boundaries with Ourselves and Others   40
He Is Waiting for Us to Surrender to Him   43
His Gift of Healing Can't Be Appropriated Until We Understand the Atonement   44
We Aren't Willing to Be Used by Him to Heal Others   46
We Think We Need to See In Order to Believe   47
Conclusion   47

Chapter 3

Why Sickness Isn't God's Plan for Our Lives 49

He Didn't Design Us for Disease 49

Healing Is Promised to Us in the Atonement 50

The Spirit Is More Effective In a Sound Mind and Body 53

In the Bible, Jesus Healed Everyone! 53

His Word Has the Power to Heal 55

Disease Is Never Called a Blessing in the Bible 58

His Name Is Jehovah-Rapha: "I Am the Lord That Heals Thee" 59

He Promises Healing in Matthew 8: 16-17 60

Jesus Said, "Greater Works than These You Shall Do" 61

Disease Blocks Us from Being Able to Do God's Work 62

God's Greater Glory Is Made Manifest When We Are Healed 64

Health Is Part of the Promise of Salvation 65

Jesus Commands Us to Heal the Sick 65

Chapter 4

A Few Reasons Why Christians Don't Believe In Miracles 67

Miracles are Rare, and Many Who Pray Don't Get One 68

Many Who Believed God for Healing Died Anyway 69

The Apostle Paul Had A "Thorn In The Flesh"—A Disease! 71

The Body Is In a Continual State of Decay 72

Chapter 5

Factors That Influence Healing and Why Some Don't Receive a Miracle 75

What Enables Healing 78

Loving Others and Providing for the Poor 78

Speaking and Meditating Upon Truth 80

Being Willing to Surrender Our Lives to Him 81

Allowing Him to Heal Us His Way, Not Ours 82

Taking Communion 84

Why We Become Blocked in Our Ability to Receive from God 85

We Don't Know How Much He Loves Us 85

Trauma Creates a False Concept of His Love 85

Subconscious Motivations Keep Us Sick 87

Disease Enables Us to Avoid Rejection and Life 87

Disease Is A Way to Get Sympathy (Love) From Others 89

We Use Disease to Punish and/or Protect Ourselves 90

Disease Is Too Comfortable 91

Disease Keeps Us from Taking Responsibility for Our Lives 93

We Are Afraid To Trust God for Good Things 94

We Feel Unworthy of God's Gift of Health 97

We Fixate on Symptoms 101

We Negate Our Faith by Our Words and Actions 103

We Harbor Unforgiveness Against Ourselves, God and Others 106

We Live in Ingratitude towards God 111

We Have a Closed Mind about God 112

Chapter 6

Where Supernatural Healing Abounds **115**

Miracles in Third-World Nations 115

Chapter 7

How to Experience the Love of God **121**

We Must See Him as a Person, Not a Religion 121

Making the Jesus of the Bible the Jesus of Our Lives 126

Hearing the Voice of God in Prayer 128

Meditating Upon His Truths 135

Knowing His Love through Images, Visions, Nature and
the Physical Touch of the Holy Spirit   137

Discovering His Love Though Prophetic Words   145

Learning About Him by "Hanging Out" With Him   148

Embracing the Power of Praise and Song   151

Walking In Obedience to Him   154

Being Sure of How He Wants To Bless Us   156

Meditating upon His Love Letter   160

Chapter 8

The Role of Satan and Our Biochemistry in
Receiving Healing from God   **167**

How Dysfunctional Brain Biochemistry Impacts Our
Relationship with God   167

The Role of Satan in Our Diseases   170

Chapter 9

The Resources That God Gave Me to Heal   **179**

Dietary Recommendations   180

Natural Hormones, Vitamins and Minerals   181

Herbs, Homeopathy, Pharmaceutical Medications and
Energy Medicine for the Treatment of Infections   183

Strategies for Removing Environmental Toxins   184

Counseling and Books   185

Physiological Strategies that Release Trauma from the Body   186

A Word of Warning about Energy Medicine   186

An Exercise for Meditating Upon the Marvel of the Body   188

How to Evaluate the Benefits of Different Healing Modalities   191

Chapter 10

To Take Medicine or Not Take Medicine

193

Chapter 11

Believing God for a Miracle

197

Appendix

The Healing Testimony of Terry Wilson

201

Bibliography   211

About the Author   215

Foreword

Healing.

It's a word that can mean very little—until your whole life depends on it. Then, that one word means the world. When you are suffering through illness, healing is something that you must hope for—to give up hope is to let the illness win. And, yet, hope is difficult: what if you have faith for healing and are disappointed? What if your hope for healing is unfounded? How are you supposed to feel hopeful when your symptoms are overwhelming? Where do you go when you *need* healing, and the ordinary world doesn't seem to help?

Healing Chronic Illness, first and foremost, is informative. The subject of supernatural—or divine—healing is clouded with confusion, misunderstanding, and myth. This balanced book brings the truth of supernatural healing to light, including how widespread it really is.

Discover why sickness isn't ultimately God's will for humanity, as well as the factors that unlock healing, as you gather resources that will enable you to receive from Him. This book will help you to learn more about His plan for healing and how that healing manifests in our modern world.

Healing Chronic Illness is filled with grace. There are no lines drawn in the sand, no shallow, one-size-fits-all remedies, and no judgments (subtle or otherwise). If you are searching for information and healing, you will be honored here.

Healing Chronic Illness is personal. In her work in the Lyme disease community, Connie Strasheim comes into contact with hundreds of chronically ill people. She never stops caring for each and every person touched by chronic illness. She tirelessly serves the chronically ill through writing and prayers, even as she struggles with symptoms herself.

Finally, this book is written by a fellow traveler. Connie is a dear friend, and I can attest: she knows what it's like to cry in desperation for a healing that has not yet arrived. And she knows what it's like to have faith for what has not yet been manifest. She knows the struggles of physical illness, as well as the financial and relational hardships that come along with that. And she is a testament of what hope really looks like, which is not, by the way, always pretty. I am astonished by her faith. And yet, as she stands in extraordinary faith, she is deeply human—which gives us all hope.

Read her story. You will receive hope here. You'll see what I mean.

Karla Johnson
Volunteer minister and counselor
Denver, Colorado

Chapter 1

God's Will for Our Wellness and What Led Me to Believe

God wants the chronically ill to be healed in body, mind and spirit. He is willing and able to heal them supernaturally when medicine fails to provide a complete recovery, and even when it doesn't. But His healing isn't always immediate, and not everyone who asks will receive a miracle.

Yet, God wants to heal more people supernaturally than are being healed today. In this book, I discuss why healing is within closer reach than what experience may have taught us to believe. I explore the reasons why physical as well as spiritual healing are God's will for humanity, and what we can do to dispel the doubts that prevent us from embracing this reality. I also describe how our dysfunctional biochemistry, unresolved emotional trauma and spiritual strongholds can hinder our knowledge of God's love for us, and consequently, our ability to receive healing from Him. I then offer solutions for addressing these and other roadblocks to healing. Finally, I ponder reasons why God may allow some to suffer prolonged illness, and how we can have faith in God for a miracle, at the same time that we reconcile ourselves to the possibility that not all of us will be fully healed on earth.

The intent of this book is to propose to the helpless and hopeless another path to wellness, which isn't based upon wishful thinking and random chance, but rather, buried truth and history, and evidence that has healed multitudes in underdeveloped nations and in Pentecostal and charismatic churches, where belief in supernatural healing is strong. A path that is less trodden in nations of wealth and reason, where reality is that which is experienced in the physical world and hope is in science and man's ability to provide. A path that is ignored because people don't know what God can do, don't realize how vast and all-encompassing His love is, and may not believe that they deserve that love, anyway. I invite you to step out and journey down this path with me. You may find that the gift of healing is meant for you, too.

I have suffered from chronic Lyme disease for over half a decade, but am receiving healing miracles in my body and spirit as I write this book. I'm also witnessing the healing of hundreds of people and being used by God to heal others. I have published two books on medical treatments for Lyme disease, and my current book is a best-seller in the Lyme disease community. Nonetheless, God has been showing me that people with Lyme and other chronic illnesses sometimes need more than medical treatments; they need a miracle. And He's showing me that He's willing and able to provide when medicine cannot.

So if you've been suffering for years from disease, why not take a chance and hope for a miracle from God? What do you have to lose? If you've invested thousands of hours and dollars into medicine, only to be frustrated by its results, losing a few months or years to a new hope may be a small sacrifice. Especially if the alternative is to continue down a path of failed or only moderately helpful treatments. Take heart—God loves you and wants to heal you!

The God of Love, the God of Miracles

So who is this God of love and miracles? Well first, He is a triune being who exists as three persons, who are all-knowing, all-powerful, and all-loving. Like you and me, these persons, known as the Father, Son and Holy Spirit, are unique in character, feelings, emotions and will, and they want to be in loving relationship with the humans that they created. The Son's name is Jesus Christ and He came to earth as a man, over 2000 years ago to show humanity what God the Father is like, and to heal and save people from their sins, since this keeps them from having a relationship with Him (more on this later). He also came to give them the Holy Spirit, who lives inside all who believe in and follow Him.

However, God speaks to everyone who seeks Him, no matter their religion, and healing miracles happen across a variety of faith systems, yet not all faith systems lead to belief in a God of love. The path of the triune God is the one I know and love, because it provides not only a complete solution to the problem of healing, but also to the problem of life and the quandary of eternity. Since this God heals in body, mind and spirit, and is the One that I have grown to love, my focus for this book will be upon Him and the hope and promises that He has given humanity, according to the Bible.

The Bible is collectively referred to as the Word of God by those who believe that its words were given by divine revelation to men in charge of communicating God's eternal truths to others. In this book, I use Jesus' teachings and Bible verses to substantiate my claims, because I believe that these teachings and verses are from God. If you aren't sure whether you believe in the Bible as the authoritative Word of God, I encourage you to study its history and ask God for a revelation of truth on the matter, because it may benefit you as you read this book.

The path of spiritual healing through the triune God; that is, through the God of Christianity and His promises in the Bible—isn't for everyone, but if I can share the gift that I have received during the eight years that I have come to know Him, I believe that some will find this gift— this deity and His promises of healing, to touch their hearts in such a manner that he becomes the solution to all that ails them. With all this in mind, in the following section, I share my personal healing journey, and the circumstances which led me to believe in miracles, and in my God's ability and willingness to heal.

My Story and the Stepping Stones of Faith

Chronic Lyme disease has disabled me for over six years. It has snatched my thirties out from under me, as most of my hours since 2004 have been devoted to sleep, tears, treatments and research for the next remedy.

Like many chronic illnesses, no cure exists in medicine for chronic (not acute) Lyme disease. The best scenario that its survivors can hope for is remission from symptoms, a place of bliss that only some attain and which isn't always permanent.

If I had known in 2004 the kind of battle that I would be up against when my body crashed overnight with an abundance of symptoms, I might have taken a different path in my healing. If I had known that my hours over the following five years would be gobbled up by arduous treatments and a never-ending search for better remedies, I might have put more of my hope in God from the beginning, and less in my treatments.

Yet I am thankful for the gains that I have made in my health since 2004. Five years on the treatment treadmill and thousands of dollars later, and I am grateful that some of my body and brain has been returned to me. I'm happy to have hints of normalcy in my daily routine, even though symptoms still clamor to be heard.

But I now know that there is sometimes a better path to wellness and God is leading me down it.

My journey down this path began after I attended the ILADS (International Lyme and Associated Diseases Society) physician's conference in October, 2009. At this conference, a prominent physician who had treated over 12,000 cases of chronic Lyme disease proclaimed that current treatments weren't working to rid most people of Babesia, one of the multiple co- infections implicated in chronic

Lyme disease. At the same time, I heard a rumor from one of the doctors that nobody ever completely gets over Lyme disease—that lifelong relapse is the reality for the afflicted. When I asked another doctor, who had treated over 11,000 patients, whether she knew of anyone who had remained in remission from Lyme disease for at least ten years, she quietly responded, "No."

Dismayed, I returned home from the conference, uncertain of which direction to take next in my healing. Having written two books on Lyme disease, I knew as much as the doctors about treatments, and sensed that I would be sentenced to the treatment treadmill for life if I hoped to maintain my healing gains. Roughly sixty to seventy percent improvement was what I had achieved and what I could keep if I continued to spend thousands of dollars and hundreds of hours per year on treatments. But was this how I wanted to live out my young adult years, which were for most healthy people my age, dedicated to dating relationships, marriage and family, recreation and getting established in a career?

Many with chronic Lyme disease, after one to five, even ten years of treatment, return to a life of relative normalcy. Thankfully, attaining an active life is possible, with the proper treatments, a strong immune system, dedication to recovery and a healthy lifestyle. But too many others, disadvantaged by trauma, unknowledgeable doctors, financial poverty or an onslaught of toxins or pathogens too fierce to overcome, struggle in the swamp of disease for decades—perhaps making gains in their healing, but still disabled by symptoms.

This battle isn't unique to those with Lyme disease; those who suffer from other chronic illnesses face similar challenges. Conventional, allopathic medicine is adept at treating many ailments. For instance, it excels in emergency medicine, but is generally confounded by the challenges of chronic illness. It tends to focus upon managing symptoms, instead of treating the underlying cause of disease. Besides, many conditions of chronic illness are difficult to heal, because they involve dysfunction in multiple bodily systems, tissues and organs, and few doctors can take the time required to address all of these. Those that do find themselves mired in a swamp of complications that requires more tools and resources than science has to offer.

Sadly, many chronic and/or degenerative diseases, such as heart disease, Crohn's, lupus, fibromyalgia, Multiple Sclerosis, cancer (which is considered to be a manageable, chronic illness in some cases), diabetes, Chronic Fatigue Syndrome, Multiple Chemical Sensitivity Syndrome, autism, Parkinson's, rheumatoid arthritis and the like, are mysteries for the medical community. Often, physicians can do no more than assign a meaningless name to the multiple systemic dysfunctions that these disorders cause and prescribe a pill or two to mitigate symptoms. The translation for these diagnoses might as well be, "The true cause behind your symptoms is unknown, so here's a label that really explains little about what's going on inside of your body."

In this book, I refer to the impact that Lyme disease has had upon my life and what it has taught me about God and healing. Yet, people suffering from other chronic diseases will be able to relate to what I share, since the symptoms of Lyme are often found in other chronic illnesses, and their impact upon a person's life is similar.

Many of the chronically ill spend their lives attempting to overcome their symptoms, or resign themselves to a life of pain, isolation and disability. Some fade from society and remain in its shadows because the fast-paced, stimulus-driven lifestyle that it demands of its participants overwhelms, and is unforgiving of those who look healthy but who can't seem to function and produce like their healthier counterparts.

I am thankful for the discoveries that have been made in medicine in recent years to help those suffering from mystery illnesses. Doctors who practice integrative and naturopathic medicine are finding solutions for the multiple dysfunctions created by chronic illness, but these solutions only partially compensate for a biochemistry gone madly awry.

Yet six years of research has made me painfully aware of what the medical community still doesn't know about disease and the body's

miraculous processes. It needs to learn much more in order to effectively combat the challenges of an increasingly toxic world, and pathogens
whose strategies for survival are outsmarting developments in medicine.

The realization that medicine probably wouldn't completely heal me
and thousands of others was one of the final catalysts that set me on a
different path to healing. In reality, though, God had started showing
me this path many months prior to ILADS.

I had been living in San Jose, Costa Rica when I first got a glimpse
of this path. Unable to work full-time, I had moved to Costa Rica from
Denver, Colorado in November, 2007, because I could no longer afford
life in the United States. I also wanted to see whether a change of
environment would accelerate my healing process.

In San Jose, Costa Rica, I attended an Assemblies of God church,
and while there, witnessed many healing miracles. I was at first skep-
tical of the bodies that would fall to the ground like a circle of
dominoes around the pulpit whenever the pastor did an altar call to heal
the broken and sick. But I soon realized that the wind of God's Spirit
was collapsing these people to the carpet and healing them, because I
once got caught up in that wind, too. A force greater than me snatched
the strength of my legs out from under me and when I fell, peace
overcame me. Sprawled about the floor, I wanted nothing more than to
take a nap amidst the pile of people around me who had also been
touched by God's Spirit.

Yet, unlike some who shared their stories of healing with me, I never got healed of my Lyme disease. That God would choose to heal my
fellow churchgoers of their hangnails and backaches but leave me
crippled by an insidious disease confounded me. I battled resentment
and bitterness against my creator. God seemed to have His favorites,
and apparently, I wasn't one of them!

"You just have to believe, Connie!" My friend José once said, rebuke threading his proclamation, as though it were my fault that I was
still sick.

Yeah, right, José. I thought bitterly. *Try believing God when you have begged Him to heal you for years but nothing ever happens!*

People prayed for my healing, time and again, and God's Spirit touched me more than once in that happy church, but it seemed that it was only to affirm His presence in my life.

Yet I learned to believe in healing miracles, because I witnessed them all around me. Once, my good friend Alejandro's face was disfigured in a car wreck and God told his mother, Roxana, also a good friend of mine, not to take her son to the plastic surgeon because He wanted to be the young man's physician. And so it was, a week after the accident, that Alejandro's face was completely healed. On another occasion, during a sermon at church, Roxana complained of having injured her back that day. Sometime during the sermon, the pastor called out, "God just healed somebody's back." Roxana, who had been sitting next to me, exclaimed excitedly, "Wow, my pain is gone! Connie, that's me!" On yet another occasion, her other son Jason was in a car wreck (yes, there are a lot of accidents in Costa Rica), and God spared him when he should have been seriously injured.

Still, since God's healing had never touched me, I didn't yet know whether supernatural healing was meant for a select few, and if God really preferred the imperfect path of medicine for a majority. Surely, He was trying to teach me something through what I was witnessing in Costa Rica!

About six months after moving back to my native city of Denver in June, 2009, I began to get more answers. Shortly after ILADS, I attended a healing conference at a church in Denver. During the conference, one woman who knew nothing about me, approached me, placed her hands upon my back and prayed for God to heal my back and central nervous system. She couldn't have known that these were my areas of greatest trouble, and I concluded that God must have revealed my problems to her because He meant to heal me. Subsequently, I received two prophecies within a month from friends who attended different churches. Both affirmed that God was healing me, but "gradually, to build my faith," which challenged my assumption that supernatural healing is always instantaneous. Further investigations led me to conclude that God can work miracles over time. One of the women who had given me a prophetic word informed me that she had been healed of a rare, incurable blood disorder, but that the healing happened seven months after she had received prayer for her condition. I felt encouraged by this.

Subsequently, I learned that my friend Troy, who also suffers from Lyme disease, was being used by God to heal people in California and Colombia. At first, the miracles were few and far between, but after awhile, the healings began to happen on a daily basis. In 2009, I traveled with him to Germany to undergo a new type of Lyme disease treatment, and while there, I noticed that he had no qualms about approaching the ailing on the street, and asking them if they wanted prayer for healing. Shortly thereafter, and after Troy traveled back to California, the miracles began to happen. God seemed to reward his boldness and willingness to pray over others by working through him to instantaneously heal others. That he was being used daily to perform miracles blew my mind.

And then, a miracle happened to me.

I had been attending another healing conference at a church in Denver called Power Invasion Ministries when God touched me. A well-known minister named Joan Hunter, who has been used by God to miraculously heal thousands, was ministering to the sick and broken. As I sat in the church, I witnessed miracle after miracle, as Joan called people down to the altar to get healed of their ailments. I thought my eyes were deceiving me when I witnessed people growing several inches in height as God replaced their vertebra and stretched out their spines, which had been compressed by injury. One woman proclaimed that she felt a tumor shrinking in her belly as Joan prayed over her, and several others were instantaneously healed of vicious maladies. A few let out shrieks and spilled tears of joy as God touched them profoundly in their bodies and spirits.

When Joan did an altar call for those needing healing from lower back pain, my heart began to race. I couldn't get to the altar fast enough.

Joan said to me, "Did you know that your right leg is two inches longer than your left?" Amazed that God had revealed this to her, I said, "Yes." She then placed her hands upon my back and as she prayed, I felt my hips and lower back shifting into a new position. The next thing I knew, she was measuring my legs and I noticed that the right one was now aligned perfectly with the left. When I returned home, I plopped down on the living room carpet with my legs extended. Normally, when I sit in this position, my right knee doesn't line up with the left, but this time, they were parallel to one another. Astounded, I also realized that I was standing differently. More of my weight had shifted to my left leg, and some of my back pain was gone. Apparently healing miracles weren't as rare as I had imagined. More importantly, I realized that God was willing to heal me, too! He wasn't blind to my suffering and wasn't withholding healing from me, just because I didn't have enough faith, as my friend in Costa Rica had insinuated. Yet the experience boosted my faith like never before.

Nearly everyone that God called to the altar that weekend seemed to receive a miracle, which further challenged my notion that God's healing is random, uncommon, and always dependent upon the faith of the recipient. In this case, it seemed to be more dependent upon the faith of the healer. In the Bible, verse 5:15 in the book of James states that, "the prayer of faith will save the sick," and many theologians interpret this verse to mean that it's the faith of the one doing the healing that counts. This fact can provide comfort to the sick when they worry that their faith is insufficient to heal them.

Yet, the faith of the one receiving healing matters, too. As I read books written by famous faith healers such as Heidi Baker, Smith Wigglesworth, Francis McNutt and FF Bosworth, I learned that greater miracles happen to those who believe in God's love and willingness to heal them.

Shortly after receiving a miracle at Power Invasion Ministries, I read FF Bosworth's book, *Christ the Healer,* which further encouraged me in my faith. Of the dozen or so books that I had read on healing, this one provided the most compelling Biblical evidence to support the theory that physical and emotional healing are gifts given to humanity because of Jesus Christ's work on the Cross, and these gifts are available to all who believe in Him. (I describe this concept more in-depth in Chapter Three). Based upon Bosworth's experiences of being used by God to heal thousands, as well as history and a plethora of Biblical evidence, rather than far-fetched suppositions, this book increased my belief in God's willingness to heal me. It also brought me tremendous joy and relief, as I realized that God not only wanted me to be healed, but that He died in order to provide me with the power that I would need in the spiritual realm to overcome my disease.

All of this newfound knowledge and experience caused me to reflect upon the ILADS conference, and the hundreds of emails and telephone calls that I had received from Lyme sufferers—people in despair because year after year of treatment had failed to cure them or they no longer had money to pay for treatments.

I doubted that God meant for health to belong only to the rich and genetically strong. Surely, He was willing to heal people of Lyme disease and other chronic illnesses by His Spirit, as He had just healed me of my back pain!

I began to ask myself some hard questions. What if the path of medicine had no end? How many more years was I, were others that I knew who struggled with chronic illness, supposed to dedicate to the pursuit of health? Did God want us to live out our days doing treatments? Surely, He was using the trial of our illnesses for our good, but it seemed wrong that He wanted us to spend year after year chasing treatments, and dedicating a majority of our waking hours to those treatments.

And the more I attended healing conferences, studied Jesus' promises and the subject of faith healing, and the more I received prophecies from others that indicated that I would be healed, the more absurd my former beliefs became.

God has created us all with a unique purpose, and it's not for us to be locked up inside of our homes, isolated from the world, with our hours and energy sucked up in the never-ending pursuit of health. We were made to love and serve others, but that task becomes complicated when disease isolates us or forces us to spend every waking minute upon our survival. I speak from experience. But in the absence of a better plan, simply abandoning the treatment treadmill and trying to survive with symptoms isn't an option for some of the chronically ill—especially if leaving the illness unattended leads to further disability.

So how many years do we do treatments in order to get better? When do we stop chasing the latest and greatest development in medicine? When I considered the absurd amount of money, time and energy that I had sunk into my healing, only to be rewarded with modest gains in my wellbeing, I realized that my life had become subject to a ruler called Lyme. And all of the treatments, instead of freeing me from my pain, had put me into bondage. They monopolized my time and thoughts, as well as my emotional, physical and financial resources, because a massive amount of everything is what's required to regain functionality from this, and many other diseases.

Not all of the chronically ill live on a treatment treadmill. They may have been told that there is no cure for their malady, so they gave up the fight long ago and decided that their disease didn't deserve that much attention. But they long for a better life. They want to participate in society; they want to be in loving relationships with others; they have dreams that they have let die because they can't "do"; and they battle depression because deep down, they know that they weren't made to hurt.

God's Plan for Our Lives

My journey has taught me that God doesn't want our lives to be filled with relentless pain, suffering and clawing at wellness. He can and will put us on a better path, if we know that path exists and are willing to walk it. My research and experiences have finally led me to take this path and to stake all of my hope for healing upon Him, because despite the risks, the path makes sense. In the following chapters, I describe other factors which have positively affected my faith and healing. May these be a source of light for you, too, and may the other concepts mentioned throughout this work provide you with hope in a loving God who heals.

Chapter 2

Why God May Allow Disease

Why would a loving God allow anyone to gimp through life slug-gishly, with pain tearing through their limbs and dysfunction preventing them from participating in society, if it were within His power to heal them? Why would such a God allow misery and depres-sion to be a part of a person's daily diet, even for years, if He could prevent it?

After all, God didn't design the body in brokenness. We are, as the Bible states in Psalm 139, "fearfully and wonderfully made." (NRSV) The problem is that the world, with all its corruption and pollution, has made a mess of our bodies so that they no longer function as God intended.

So, assuming that God is sovereign and that by praying according to His will, "…we know that we have obtained the requests made of him" (1 John 5:15, NRSV), and that He can heal supernaturally, then why aren't all who seek healing made well? In churches where healing miracles happen, why do some get healed, while others must walk away without their miracle?

Despite the fact that God works miracles and wants us to be well, He sometimes allows disease for a short (or long!) season, and not always because we lack faith! Discussion of the reasons why this happens is important for remaining encouraged as we look to Him for healing, and in the following sections, I describe what some of those reasons are.

Our Faith Is in Medicine

Even the chronically ill who believe in miracles usually trod the difficult path of medicine, and spend endless dollars and hours on therapies and drugs designed to keep them functional and/or alive. The treatments are a buffer to their suffering and may enable them to live a more functional life than they otherwise would, but are rarely a complete solution to their maladies. Still, they often end up inadvertently putting their faith in this imperfect medicine instead of in God, because His miracles seem reserved for a select few. Some resign themselves to a life of limited functionality or find peace in their disability as they rely upon the resources that God has provided them in the natural world to get by.

Those who don't believe that miracles are one of God's favorite methods for healing the sick argue that He gave us doctors and healers, plants, drugs, herbs and vitamins for wellness. He gave us brains with which to develop cures for disease, and, hasn't all this stuff proven to help humanity more than hope in some random God who occasionally does miracles? The things of the natural world seem to be more reliable to them, since they can go to the doctor, get a pill for this or that ailment, and chances are, it will make them well. Or they believe that God will guide them to the right place to get the right drug. They believe that few people receive miracles, and that those who had faith in God for healing but who died anyway—are sore but solid proof that we can't rely upon Him to be made well.

The remedies that God has provided on earth for our healing are a miracle in and of themselves. Herbs work wonders to heal the body.

Surgeries save lives. Insulin keeps diabetics alive, and God uses all of these things to make people well. And for those who don't believe in God, they are their only hope. But even those who believe in a God of miracles often feel safer pursuing remedies in the natural world, than asking their Creator to heal them supernaturally.

In the Bible, Jesus said that we need to have faith in Him (and the Father) if we want to receive from Him. Chapter 11, verse 6 in the book of Hebrews states: "And without faith, it is impossible to please God, for whoever would approach Him must believe that He exists and that He rewards those who seek him." But if our hope is in medicine more than in God, then He may not be able to heal us, out of respect for our free will. If we have been conditioned by experience to believe that there is a greater likelihood of being made well by a drug than by God, then our hope will be set upon the drug, not Him. While we may argue that our ultimate hope is in Him, medicine or no medicine, in order to have faith for a miracle, we must know that supernatural healing can happen as commonly as healing through medicine. And when we are healed by medicine, we must realize that it is only because God has blessed it.

By Our Trials We Are Ultimately Made Well

Some ministers of charismatic and Pentecostal churches contend that God doesn't allow disease in order to teach His people a lesson. They argue that such a belief is punishing, and causes people to con-clude that they are sick because they have done something wrong. But if we don't know that God wants us to be well, then perhaps the lesson is simply for us to learn that He loves us and is willing to heal us! That lesson isn't always learned overnight, but we may not be able to receive healing in our bodies and spirits until we understand this. Thankfully, the Holy Spirit guides us into all truth and will help us to embrace God's truths if we seek Him.

In my healing journey, whenever I have prayed and asked God what I need to do in order to be well, His still, quiet voice always tells me the same thing; that He wants me to be healed in my physical body, but more importantly, He wants me to be whole. And if the journey through disease ultimately brings me to a place of wholeness, then I must trudge through it. Wholeness means perfect health in body, mind and spirit, and sometimes, He requires the participation of my will to achieve that.

Healing can't always happen through a simple wave of His holy hand. In the process that leads to wholeness, the will, emotions and thoughts must all be involved, so the ultimate healing of body, mind and spirit can take time. This is especially true in the chronically ill, whose symptoms are often caused, at least in part, by emotional trauma. God sometimes needs us to work with Him to heal this trauma, if our bodies and minds are to be fully healed. We may, for instance, need to learn to think and speak life-giving words to ourselves and others, which is a discipline that, once learned and effectively practiced, leads to health. Evidence for this is found in the book of Proverbs. Chapter 12, verse 18 states that: "...the tongue of the wise brings healing." Similarly, Proverbs 16:24 states, "Pleasant words are like a honeycomb, sweetness to the soul and health to the body."

I wonder if those who believe that God doesn't allow disease for good and to ultimately make us whole have ever experienced a prolonged period of illness—as in, many months or years. While I don't believe that God ultimately wants us to live out our entire lives in pain and fatigue (for reasons that I will discuss in the following chapters), my experience has taught me that it's a fallacy that disease can't be used as a powerful teacher and catalyst for spiritual growth and healing.

Sickness Forces Us to Face Our Demons

Living with illness has a funny way of forcing us to face the demons of our past head-on. Years of studying medicine has taught me that unresolved emotional trauma plays a significant role in the development of physical disease. The unhealed who have tried dozens of remedies often suffer from this problem. Yes, they may have pathogens and toxins aplenty sucking the life out of their limbs, but it's the emotional ghosts which allow those toxins to stay there, unless they get healed from their trauma.

When I got sick, I realized that I had no choice but to face my phantoms or remain mired in the muck of disease. It's impossible to heal from chronic illness when there are big, scary ghosts in your closet. I have discovered this to be true for others who suffer from chronic illness, as well.

Because Lyme left me isolated in my home for months, with no job and little to do but treatments, it was easier for me to face these demons because I no longer had the distractions of work, an active social life and recreational activities to keep me occupied. My healing process involved more than just taking an anti-depressant, which is the convenient, fast solution for busy people who can't, or won't, take the time to pray, seek counseling or research other methods for healing. But healing emotional trauma is usually a complicated matter, not easily resolved by medication, weekly sessions with a therapist, or ten hurried minutes of prayer at the end of the night. For me, none of these interventions, in and of themselves, would have been sufficient. I needed hours of grief processing time with God; more hours dedicated to receiving help from my life's mentors, and years to meditate upon and learn how to change my harmful beliefs and thinking patterns.

When it comes to healing emotional trauma, in the chronically ill, the stakes are high. We may have no choice but to face our ghosts or remain physically ill. Fortunately, disability and disease can provide us with the time and motivation to resolve issues that we might have otherwise ignored for years.

Sickness Teaches Us How to Develop Healthy Habits

Disease can also challenge us to re-think our life's activities and adopt healthier eating and other habits. For example, when I got sick with Lyme, I realized that I could no longer afford to fuel my body with refined food and sugar. Neither could I afford to live life at the same breakneck pace as before. Toxic food and a rushed lifestyle had contributed to the breakdown of my body, and I soon learned that becoming pals with salad and salmon would be vital for my recovery. God showed me that this was the kind of food that He had made the body to thrive on, and I would live longer and better on a diet of greens, unrefined carbohydrates, and antibiotic and hormone-free animal protein, no matter my physical condition. Eighty percent of the food sold in supermarkets today is canned, boxed and/or processed. Such food is virtually nutrient-less and contains many added chemicals that poison the body. No wonder the rate of chronic disease is climbing, but I would have scarcely paid attention to the problem of fake food had it not been for Lyme disease.

Most of the chronically ill can't afford to eat whatever they want. A daily doughnut can leave them permanently camping on the sofa, while a healthy, nutrient-rich diet enables them to remain relatively functional. Because of their vulnerability to symptoms, many of the sick shun pasta, sugary bread and all of the processed food that healthier people can tolerate. The discipline to eat right is easier when consuming healthy foods becomes a question of life or death. Fortunately, those who learn to eat well often resolve to never go back to their old ways, because illness has taught them that eating the right stuff matters. So God may allow disease if it teaches us to change our eating habits, because this may be what ultimately brings us the greatest health over the long haul. Our bodies are His creation, as well as the temple of His Holy Spirit, and He wants us to treat them well. In the Bible, 1 Corinthians 6:19-20 states: "Or do you not know that your body is a temple of the Holy Spirit within you, which you have from God, and that you are not your own? For you were bought with a price; therefore, glorify God in your body."

Illness can teach us to adopt other healthy habits as well, which may be just as important as a proper diet. Before I became sick, I used to rush through life at an anxious pace in an effort to accomplish always more. This thrust my body into a continual "fight or flight" response that drained my adrenal glands and kept me from enjoying the roses. Stopping and smelling them had never been part of my existence, because I had lived under the lie that many fall prey to—that greater productivity leads to increased happiness, acceptance and self- importance. We feel good about ourselves when we get things done. Our society values production, results, doing and more doing…but there is always a higher ladder to climb and more to be done. The drive to produce becomes a drug as addictive as any other, but letting go of the drug is painful, because it means that the place where we have stashed our self-worth gets snatched out from under us. While I haven't yet learned to be content in just being instead of doing, I don't dash through life like before, because now, I simply can't. I pay too high a price for it. One day of rushing and doing at breakneck speed renders me useless the following day. So there's no point.

I have spoken with many chronically ill who bemoan that they can no longer accomplish as much as when they were healthy. Life seems like a waste, and while disease squanders their productivity, they will admit that the positive side to this is that they have stopped trying to find their worth in what they do, because they can't. They must look within to discover new sources of happiness and self-worth. Fortunately, many end up finding it within the spiritual realm and in a relationship with God. They also learn that rushing around and living life in the fast lane doesn't necessarily lead to greater happiness, but instead depletes the body, soul and spirit.

So God may allow us to be sick for a time, if, in our sickness, we learn to adopt new lifestyle habits. Because if sleeping four hours per night and living on fast-forward is what caused us to get sick in the first place, we must change the way that we approach life before we can be healed and remain that way. Again, it's about glorifying and treating properly what God has made!

Sickness Teaches Us Dependence upon Him

God can use our battles with illness to teach us to depend upon Him for all of our needs. In my life, I learned that one of the byproducts of chronic illness is financial devastation. Unable to work and facing incredible health care costs, the chronically ill often survive on crumbs. Since 2004, I have spent an average of $1,500 per month, sometimes more, on supplements, drugs, doctor visits and other therapies to stay afloat and functional. To survive the onslaught of medical expenses, I have had to rely upon God to provide for me in unexpected ways. It hasn't been easy but it has taught me humility and to lean upon Him instead of myself. It's a fallacy that we have control over our lives, and poverty is a prime opportunity for us to relinquish control over our money. When devastated by medical bills and an inability to work, no other choice remains but to trust God to provide, even if His methods of provision elude us.

 A good friend of mine, whom I will call Sarah (to protect her identity), suffers from a severely disabling manifestation of Lyme disease. She was abandoned by her husband after becoming ill. Too sick to work, she now relies solely upon the charity of others to survive. There are times when she doesn't know how she will pay for groceries, yet somehow, money always turns up. God provides because she has learned to trust that He will come through for her, even though that provision sometimes arrives last-minute.

When we are functional and able to work a steady job, we tend to rely less upon God, and more upon our own ability to bring in a paycheck. We may know that He's our ultimate provider, but when we lose the ability to work, we look to Him more closely to meet our needs. Philippians 4:19 says: "And my God will fully satisfy every need of yours according to His riches in glory in Christ Jesus." Everything we have comes from Him and only Him, and we realize this in greater measure when our ability to provide for ourselves gets snatched out from under us. Receiving His provision when the odds are stacked against us also strengthens our trust in Him, as we learn that He desires to, and can, provide for all that we need, no matter our circumstances.

Thus, God may allow illness for a time, if it teaches us to depend upon Him, because such dependence may be what we need for a lifetime of spiritual health.

Before I got sick, I believed in God, but didn't have a personal relationship with Him. Getting sick forced me to realize how much I needed Him. Sadly, I would not have been willing to turn my life over to Him had this not happened to me. Because I did, I ended up receiving the greatest healing in the world—His love, and consequently, greater emotional and spiritual health.

Sickness Motivates Us to Change Our Thoughts

If we are receptive, God can use chronic illness to motivate us to change our thoughts and become more positive people. Biochemical dysfunction and a life of isolation conspire fiercely against the ability to remain joyful and positive, but it doesn't serve the sick to live in despondency and sadness any more than it serves the healthier soul. This, of course, doesn't mean that the sick aren't entitled to their tears and pessimism. Living with disease for years steals hope and happiness from the heart, and it can be a herculean feat to believe God for a better life when year after year, nothing changes. It may be even more difficult to find the good in a life that can accomplish so little, especially if that life must be lived alone.

Indeed, in my sicker days, I used to snap off heads whenever well-meaning friends or family would admonish me to "just be a little more positive." My back hurt. I couldn't think. Anxiety gripped me at every turn. My bowels didn't function. My heart raced. I got weak while standing in line. I couldn't breathe. I spent most of my waking hours alone because I was unable to work. My friends spent their energy and money on recreational activities that I couldn't participate in, so instead of joining them in their fun, I threw myself pity parties. With lots of whine and cheese!

Also, during the first years that I suffered from Lyme disease, my neurological dysfunction was severe. Depression caused me to despair over my circumstances and cry for no apparent reason. I saw the world through darkly tinted lenses. It seemed that everybody was out to get me and nobody cared that I was dying (apparently!).

Yet, I realized that my symptoms, isolation, and all the rest could easily become a crutch and an excuse to wallow in the muck and over time, I learned not to stay there because it didn't benefit me. We may be entitled to our despondency, and shooing it away requires massive effort when our symptoms clamor to be heard, but living in dark thoughts is almost a guarantee that we won't make it out of the mess of chronic illness.

It's not fair, is it? Living with a positive mindset is difficult enough when the body functions relatively well, but when the biochemistry of the brain is a mess, such a feat can seem impossible. Fortunately, all things are possible with God's Spirit, if we know that a power greater than our biochemistry lives within us.

This Spirit can teach us to be joyful in all circumstances, and help us to change our negative thoughts, which is an integral part of the healing puzzle. While disease conspires against positive thinking, the Spirit can motivate us to develop the habit of meditating upon all that is lovely and precious about life, because our healing might be contingent upon us finding the sterling in the storm cloud. We may have more time to ponder that silver lining, anyway, if we can't do much more than pad around our apartments. Besides, when disease has stolen away opportunities for happiness within the worldly realm, the only other place where it can be found is in the mind and spirit. And if we can learn to manage our thoughts amidst the storms of illness, then we can be masters at managing them throughout all of life's circumstances. This may prevent another illness from striking us ten years down the road. When the thoughts are right, then the rest of life goes right. God once showed me that He could heal my physical body right now, but as long as my thoughts remained a mess, I would be prone to disease.

Sometimes, chronic illness creates such mental dysfunction and de-pression that nothing short of a miracle from God and the prayers of others will heal our thoughts. At other times, God may allow illness if He knows it will motivate us to change our thinking. Such changes may be what we need for a lifetime of wellness, because people who live in a state of constant negativity and who disbelieve God's promises don't tend to stay healthy.

During the first few years of my illness, I suffered from so much mental dysfunction that it was difficult for me to control my thoughts. As I healed my brain with medicine, I found that I was increasingly able to exercise self-control and choose what I wanted to think. Subsequently, God began to teach me how to affirm His promises and speak His truths, so that I would become receptive to His love and to receiving a greater healing miracle. If I had remained sick and stuck in my pessimism, I might not have been able to receive those promises, because in my depression, it was incredibly difficult to believe that He wanted to heal me. So I had to heal my brain and then allow Him to teach me to think differently.

In the following chapters, I provide suggestions for healing the brain and strategies for changing your thoughts, so that you may be better equipped to receive a deeper healing from God.

Only Those Who Have "Been There, Suffered That" Are Qualified to Empathize with the Sick

Some people battle the challenges of disease and disability on their own. Their family and friends mysteriously vanish when they become ill, because they can't handle their grief, are too wrapped up in their own lives, or don't believe that their loved ones are really *that* sick. They may also feel helpless, and so avoid them out of sadness, guilt or fear. The chronically ill often look stellar on the outside, but are shredded on the inside. So they are labeled hypochondriacs, judged for their apparent laziness, and left bereft of sorely needed emotional and financial support. Or maybe they do wear a wan complexion and raccoon eyes, but even their most compassionate friend can't fathom the suffering that they face daily, and provide the support that they need. They may be fed unhelpful advice, as loved ones admonish them to get a job, brighten their outlook, or seek better solutions for their healing. It isn't uncommon for friends and family to have only a vague awareness of the needs of the chronically ill, no matter how hard they try to comprehend their challenges. Words just don't suffice, and only souls who have worn the shoes of infirmity can empathize with the sick and know what they need. One of the worst things that well-meaning Christian peers can do to their loved ones is accuse them of not having enough faith to be healed, or judge them for not having enough godly joy in their lives. Sometimes, only the godly who have "been there, suffered that" have the necessary grace and wisdom to offer to the sick. Sometimes, what the sick need most is for someone to sit with them in silence or hold them in their tears. Those who can empathize or relate to their suffering are most qualified to do this and provide them with the love that they need.

This leads to one of the greatest arguments for why God may allow chronic illness. Because the sick need more than sympathy; they need empathy, and only those who have "been there, suffered that" can provide that. They need people who truly know what it's like to awaken day after day in vicious pain or with fatigue and brain fog, with no reprieve for years. Such people can usually offer a higher level of compassion for their suffering and tend to have a greater understanding of their needs.

The work of Lyme-literate physicians represents a perfect example of how God allows the sicknesses of some to help others through their suffering. Most doctors in the United States don't know how to adequately treat chronic Lyme disease, because the politics behind the disease have prevented them from receiving proper education or training about it. (For more information on the politics of Lyme, read Pamela Weintraub's best-selling book, *Cure Unknown*). Yet it is documented to be the fastest-growing infectious disease in the United States, with an estimated 200,000 cases (or more) every year. Extraordinarily complicated and expensive to treat, and because of the politics surrounding diagnosis and treatment, those physicians that know how to adequately treat chronic Lyme are being actively persecuted by medical boards and the powers that be for their efforts to heal others. This means that the only doctors who are willing to risk treating Lyme patients are (usually) those that have suffered through the disease themselves, or who have somebody in their family who has. They comprehend its brutal reality, and out of compassion, want to save others from the hell that they themselves went through, no matter the personal cost. Few doctors who haven't experienced Lyme would ever take that risk or be willing tackle the difficulties of treating it.

Disease Motivates Us to Advance Our Knowledge of Medicine to Heal Others

God may also allow disease if it sparks the development of new remedies in medicine. Medicine is imperfect but God also uses it to heal people, especially those who don't believe in miracles. Nothing drives research like desperation, especially when no cure has yet been found for a disease. Because I was unfortunate enough (or fortunate enough!) to have been struck by a disease that most of the medical community is ignorant about, I realized that I would have to find my own way out of the mess of Lyme (because at the time of my diagnosis, there were no Lyme-literate physicians in Colorado, where I lived). This required countless hours of research, until I had amassed enough information to write a book on the subject. So when I had written and published two books on Lyme just four years into my healing journey, I realized that God had indeed used my trial for good, because now I could provide thousands with the tools that they would need to treat their Lyme disease in the realm of medicine. As imperfect as these tools are, they have served to relieve many of their suffering. Never would I have become a medical writer if it hadn't been for Lyme disease, so who knows if God didn't allow my suffering so that thousands of others would be helped?

As another example, I know several naturopathic doctors who chose their profession because they once suffered from chronic illness and conventional medicine failed to cure them. Because naturopathic medicine focuses upon treating the cause of disease, not its symptoms (as conventional western medicine often does), it is usually better at treating chronic conditions. Knowing this, some doctors of naturopathic medicine became motivated to choose their career path because of their own prior suffering. So God may allow illness for a time if it enables us to advance our medical knowledge and heal others through what we have learned.

Disease Teaches Us to Set Healthy Boundaries with Ourselves and Others

Another important reason why God may allow sickness is so that we learn to set healthier boundaries with ourselves and others. Essentially, boundaries are dividing lines between us and everyone else that represents both the physical and emotional limits that we may not violate in one another. They define our sense of self and teach us what our responsibilities towards ourselves and others should be.

For example, people who can't say "no" to others have weak boundaries. When this happens, their bodies will often express that "no" for them in the form of symptoms. When people don't refuse abuse; always accede to the demands and wishes of others; fail to express their needs or dishonor themselves by not living true to their values and who they are, then resentment builds and their bodies swallow that bitter pill.

Before I crashed with an abundance of symptoms in 2004, I had been working fourteen-hour days as a Flight Attendant for United Airlines, and while I knew that such long workdays were too much for my body to handle long-term, I ignored the voice of my conscience that was pleading with me to take a different direction in my career. Physically exhausted, I continued to push myself beyond my body's ability to handle the work, and sure enough, one day, it was as if my body said, "No more!", and the Lyme bugs, which had up until then been kept under wraps by my immune system, came out to play.

Many people have had their voices silenced throughout their lives, by abusive caretakers, spouses, or others in authority. When this happens in childhood, particularly, the damage can be far-reaching and severe. If your parents or caretakers ridiculed or punished you for having an opinion; if you were harmed or silenced for expressing your needs; belittled, ignored, or in some other way taught that your needs didn't matter to those in charge of your livelihood, you would have, consciously or subconsciously, resented those who denied you the ability to express yourself. But even though you couldn't express the resentment, rage, fear and sadness that would have resulted from such trauma—those emotions still had to go somewhere. Chances are, you internalized them, where they festered and grew inside of you, until one day, they made you sick or contributed to the breakdown of your body.

While ignoring my body's need for rest contributed to its break-down, I also became sick because I hadn't been living true to myself in other areas of my life. Since childhood and up until my "breakdown" with Lyme disease in 2004, I had often repressed my feelings, thoughts and opinions (essentially, my "true self")—out of fear of what others would think of or do to me. While I harbored Lyme infections in my body for years before becoming sick, those infections were allowed to become active because I had a lifelong track record of silencing my voice in moments when I should have expressed myself. Because I didn't say "no" to people who took advantage of me; because I complied with others' wishes and requests out of fear instead of love, and because I stuffed my thoughts and emotions, I secretly resented others, and my body stored that resentment in the form of symptoms. Fortunately, many years spent studying books on the concept of boundaries, as well as counseling and prayer, have since helped me to develop a stronger sense of self. They have taught me how to identify abusive behaviors and situations and say "no" to those. It has taken me a long time to learn that true love isn't about being compliant and agreeable; it's about being honest, with myself and others.

The concept of boundaries encompasses so much more than just living true to ourselves, however. Because this subject is so broad, I encourage you to read the *Boundaries* book series by Drs. Cloud and Townsend, in order to better identify how a lack of boundaries may be contributing to your lack of physical and emotional health.

Also, it's important to mention that some people suffer from disease not only because they aren't able to set boundaries with themselves and others today, but also because someone forcefully violated their boundaries in the past—and either they didn't know that they were being violated or they couldn't do anything about it (as in cases of child abuse or rape). Healing from the effects of such violations upon our bodies and psyches requires a more comprehensive approach than simply learning to set boundaries with others. It requires counseling, prayer and medical interventions to heal the body, mind and spirit (more on these in the following chapters).

Fortunately, people who suffer from chronic illness often develop a keen sense for when their boundaries are being violated, because their bodies let them know through an exacerbation of symptoms that something is wrong. Having this awareness may motivate them to avoid unhealthy behaviors, stressful situations and toxic relationships because they realize that these will further damage their health. So symptoms serve as a kind of radar for when they are in an abusive or damaging relationship with another, or when they are doing something that is harmful to their well-being.

Thus, God may allow illness for a time, if it helps us to take a long, hard look at the ways in which we are dishonoring ourselves and others in relationships. Once we do this, we can then learn new ways to constructively express who we are instead of repressing the voice of our conscience—indeed, of God.

Finally, establishing boundaries with others isn't selfish. It's about being honest and true to ourselves; a lesson that a loving God would want His people to learn. Asking God through prayer to reveal the ways in which we dishonor ourselves and others is a good idea. The Holy

Spirit will reveal to us our unhealthy lifestyle habits and relational patterns, if we ask Him to and are willing to receive His truths with a humble spirit. Once we have these truths, He will empower and embolden us to establish healthier relationships, with the help of godly mentors and counselors.

He Is Waiting for Us to Surrender to Him

God is keen on surrender because the only way that His life can flow through us is if we submit our wills to Him and learn to trust Him above our own intelligence. When we let go of doing life our way, He can then move in us to do things His way. The process of letting go may be agonizing, because we are hurt and broken humans who are, understandably, afraid of letting go of our way of "doing life" because it feels safe to us (even though it may not be!). Yet God's ways always bring about greater peace than ours, and He may allow difficult trials, such as disease, to get us to give up and turn to Him for guidance, wisdom and all that we need for the abundant life that He has promised us. Because when man's medicine fails us, our bank accounts are empty, and all goes awry, it's much easier for us to throw up our hands and say, "Well, okay God, my way isn't working, so let's try Yours!" It's a blessing in disguise, even though while we go through it, all we see is the ugly disguise.

Surrender is also facilitated when all of life's goodies get snatched out from under us, as often happens when we get whacked by disease. We lose important relationships and material possessions, as well as the ability to work and participate in society. What remains after the whole world has left us, but a God who will keep us company? Embracing Him is sometimes the only alternative to insanity, and so we do it. It's sad that this is what it takes for us to acknowledge our God, who so deeply loves us, but when we do, we discover the greatest source of peace and wisdom that we have ever known. The discovery doesn't happen overnight. It may take a year, or two, or twenty, before we understand that the gift of a relationship with Him is the greatest gift in the world. But He promises that we will find Him when we search after Him with all of our heart and soul. (Deuteronomy 4:29)

Ultimately, the promise of eternal life and God's love are the most important gifts that we can receive on earth, so if sickness is the only way that He can bring our attention to these greater gifts, He may allow it for a time, because being in a surrendered, loving relationship with Him *is* the ultimate expression of health. Often, it is this relationship that eventually heals the body, too.   As previously mentioned, I wouldn't have decided to follow God had I not become ill.   But now I wouldn't trade my relationship with God for a life of total physical health. I have learned by experience that His love is the most important thing in the world; far more valuable than gold, popularity or a body that functions properly. The wisdom, peace and self-acceptance that He has given me, and which I would have never discovered without Him, are priceless.   They have enabled me to live a happier, healthier life of greater purpose, and to prosper in my relationships with others. Without the ability to love and be loved by others, life is meaningless, and my relationship with God has increased my capacity to give and receive love, in ways that I could not before I knew Him.

His Gift of Healing Can't Be Appropriated Until We Understand the Atonement

Authors of books that refute supernatural healing cite many reasons why they believe that God doesn't perform healing miracles today, or why they believe such miracles are scarce. Like the authors of these books, I don't believe that everyone who asks for a miracle will receive one, but my conviction is that He wants all of us to be well. Unlike the skeptics, however, my research and experience have taught me that God wants to and is performing more healing miracles than many of us realize. I also believe that spiritual, emotional, mental and physical healing were given to us as a gift, because of Jesus Christ's atoning work on the Cross—that is, when Jesus took our sins upon himself and died on a Cross over 2000 years ago, he also took our sicknesses, as well (the Atonement is explained in Chapter 5). But perhaps this gift can only be appropriated to the degree that we walk in submission to God's Spirit and know that we have received healing just as surely as we have received His gift of salvation which leads to eternal life. Those who have a greater experience and understanding of God's love and what Christ's sacrifice has provided for them may experience more miracles.

That said, God sometimes heals as a demonstration of His love, regardless of our knowledge of Him and our standing in Jesus Christ. Recently, I attended a four-day healing school, hosted by Global Awakening ministries. At this school, one of the teachers, Randy Clark, a minister who has been used by God to heal thousands worldwide, shared that non-Christians often receive more healing miracles than Christians. He said that God sometimes uses those who don't even believe in divine healing to heal others, and that the ungodly often receive more miracles than the godly. He went on to say that this is to demonstrate that all of God's gifts are given to us by His grace, not by our works. In the Bible, Ephesians 2:8 states that, "For by grace you have been saved through faith, and this is not your own doing, it is the gift of God". Imagine if we could attain healing by our works! We would risk becoming prideful and arrogant and strive to receive the gift of healing by our own efforts instead of by His Spirit. That God uses the unbeliever and the unholy to heal and be healed is a powerful demonstration of His grace and love towards all humanity. There is nothing we can do to become more acceptable to Him. It is only by His Spirit that we are able to do anything that He may require of us to be made well.

Randy Clark also believes that one reason why non-Christians tend to be healed more often than Christians is because many Christians have been taught that God doesn't heal the sick anymore, and that Jesus' sacrifice on the Cross was only meant to save us from our sins. But sickness is to the body what sin is to the soul. These Christians' minds are full of theological roadblocks that God must remove before they can be made well. But, if they, if we, are willing, He will revamp our beliefs and reveal to us the full meaning of the Atonement, which provides solid proof of His willingness and ability to heal us .

We Aren't Willing to Be Used by Him to Heal Others

The manifestation of God's healing miracles doesn't depend solely upon His willingness to heal, but also upon our willingness to be used by Him to perform these miracles. Who knows if millions are sick because we aren't willing to step out and pray for those who are struggling along in the streets or dying in hospital beds? God sometimes works independently of His people, but most of the time, we are the preferred instruments that He uses to carry out His will. So if we aren't bold enough to lay hands on our hurting neighbor whenever the Spirit whispers, "Hey, that guy over there could use a little prayer," then that poor soul may remain ill. This is one reason why we don't witness an abundance of miracles in our society—because of the sad, simple fact of our unwillingness to pray. Imagine if every one of us laid hands on and prayed for just one sick person per day! How many fewer people would we lose to disease if, in faith, we stepped out and followed Jesus' command to pray for and heal the sick? In the Bible, James 5:15 states: "The prayer of faith will save the sick." Verse 16 continues this idea: "Therefore, confess your sins to one another, and pray for one another, so that you may be healed."

So what about the poor and destitute in Africa and other places who aren't aware that God heals? Well, God does many miracles in Africa, but Africa also needs the bigger miracles of food, water and disease prevention, if the people in its poorest nations are to remain well. Since God uses His people to meet the needs of others, if we refuse to provide so that people in Africa and other nations can build water wells and buy mosquito nets, then on some level, it won't matter how many healing miracles the people receive, because filarial worms in the water supply or a malarial bug will simply take them down again the following day, week or month. At the same time, we must be willing to travel to these destitute places and allow God to work in the hearts and bodies of the people there, if they are to be healed. Then maybe there wouldn't be so many millions of sick and the world would learn to believe that God still does miracles today.

We Think We Need to See In Order to Believe

I once heard Joan Hunter say at a healing conference that healing miracles are more common than most people realize, but those who haven't witnessed any tend to think they are rare. Some of us need to see in order to believe, yet God admonishes us to believe before we see. In John 20:29, Jesus says, "Blessed are those who have not seen and yet have come to believe." Throughout the Bible, God asks His people to believe in order to receive His gifts.

When we have never seen a healing miracle, believing that they are common may be difficult for us. It can take our image and expectations of God too far outside of the realm of our experience. Yet, if we open our hearts and minds to the possibility that God can accomplish "abundantly far more than all we can ask or imagine" (Ephesians 3:20), and choose to believe in His promises of healing even before we see their manifestation, we will receive from Him. We may have to persevere for awhile, but if we continue to hold onto His truths, those promises will eventually manifest. If we require evidence before we will believe God for anything, however, then we may remain ill until we decide to embrace His way of doing things—which means deciding to believe Him for our healing before we see or feel it.

In Conclusion

All of the above represent a sampling of the reasons, based on my experience, why God may allow disease. Ironically, all of these reasons are linked to God's desire to ultimately heal, in body, mind and spirit, as well as to our day-to-day decision to cooperate with Him and trust Him in the process. If these reasons are valid, then it isn't truly His will for anyone to remain sick, but He may allow sickness for a season, until we learn the beliefs and behaviors that are necessary for receiving and maintaining health.

Depending upon how you see it, this can be a scary thought that makes receiving health dependent upon your performance. Or it can be an encouragement, if we know that God will create the changes in us by His power, as long as we are willing to acknowledge and surrender to Him with a humble heart.

Perhaps there are other reasons why God allows disease. After all, who can know His mind? While we will never know all of the reasons why God allows illness, I believe that, with His help, we can learn to trust Him and believe in His promises, anyway. He is the healer, and ultimately, works all things together for our good, even though we may not understand what that "good" is at the time.

Chapter 3

Why Sickness Isn't God's Plan for Our Lives

He Didn't Design Us for Disease

Well, for starters, God didn't originally create the human body to be sick or broken. That some of us were born broken or sick doesn't mean that this was part of God's original design process. We may live in a fallen world, but the Holy Spirit still operates within it and fixes some of humanity's messes. The amount of work that He can do in us, however, often depends upon our willingness to cooperate with Him. If and when we do, He heals our bodies that have been tattered and battered by the world or in the womb. If God loves us, and His original design for the body is health, then common sense dictates that if He can restore us, He will! If it were within your power to heal your sick child, would you not do it? How much more will God, who loves us infinitely more than our earthly parents, heal His children!

Healing Is Promised to Us in the Atonement

Christ the Healer, among other excellent books on supernatural healing, provides concrete Biblical evidence that physical healing was one of God's promises to all who would accept Jesus Christ's atoning sacrifice and receive the Holy Spirit. The book is compelling because its arguments are based on Biblical truths and history, rather than some preacher's whimsical suppositions or man's faulty wisdom.

The Old Testament books of the Bible provide over 300 predictions regarding Jesus Christ's life and ministry on earth, all of which were fulfilled in the New Testament. These predictions provide some of the most compelling evidence that the Bible is inspired by God and that healing was given to us because of Jesus Christ's work on earth, and especially, His death on the Cross.

Isaiah was the Bible's most important Old Testament prophet. He lived around 680 BC, nearly 700 years before Jesus Christ came to earth, and made many predictions regarding His birth, life and ministry. That every one of his prophecies was fulfilled nearly 700 years later testifies to the truthfulness of his words. The original Biblical scrolls that we have today and which contain Isaiah's prophecies date back to approximately 150 BC and the predictions in the scrolls are the same as those published in Bibles today, so they are thought to be accurate. The Dead Sea Scrolls discovery in 1958 also helped to confirm their accuracy.

One of Isaiah's prophecies describes Jesus Christ's atoning work on the Cross, and the redemptive promises that humanity would receive through His death and resurrection. These promises are described in Isaiah 53:3-5. I believe that the New Revised Standard Version of the Bible provides one of the most accurate translations of these verses, because it is based on ancient manuscripts that were discovered after the King James Bible was published (which has been, historically, the most accepted version of the Bible). Because of these manuscripts, scholars discovered defects in the King James translation, and therefore, produced a more revised, updated version of the Bible to reflect what they discovered—hence the NRSV.   Isaiah 53:3-5, in the NRSV version reads:

> "He (Jesus) is despised, and rejected by others;
> A man of suffering and acquainted with infirmity (some versions of the Bible inaccurately translate "infirmity" as "grief")
> And as one from whom others hide their faces
> He was despised, and we held him of no account
> Surely he has borne our infirmities and carried our diseases;
> Yet we accounted him stricken, struck down by God, and afflicted.
> But he was wounded for our transgressions,
> Crushed for our iniquities;
> Upon him was the punishment that made us whole,
> And by his bruises we are healed."

These verses describe Jesus' suffering on the Cross and how He bore the punishment for our sins and sicknesses there, so that we could be healed and fully reconciled to God, once and for all. He literally took all of our sin upon Himself in His body, suffering what we should have suffered for our sin (or estrangement from God). The verses also describe our attitude towards Him; how we despised Him and deemed Him insignificant and unworthy of praise, instead of as our wonderful Savior who brings us back to our Father.

Jesus' sacrifice atoned for every mess that humanity has ever made, and will ever make. If we acknowledge that act and realize that a heavy price must be paid for our sin, and if we choose to repent; that is, turn away from doing life our way and instead embrace His way, then He promises to forget about every bad thing that we have ever done to Him, ourselves and others. He erases from His memory every evil word, wicked glance, and hateful act that we have ever committed against our brother, sister and selves, and instead, sees us through a lens of perfection; as Christ himself, in our flesh.

Because of Jesus' work on the Cross, God heals us and His Spirit comes to live in us and through us—if we invite Him in. Through Him, we become empowered to live a holy, joyous life, because the same

Spirit that lived in Jesus and which raised Him from the dead now lives in us. Like Jesus, we are given the power to perform miracles, which we appropriate as the Spirit dictates and according to God's perfect will. Sadly, many people have this power but are unaware of it or suppress it through unbelief or a decision to continue to do life their way, instead of God's way, because they don't want to submit to anyone or anything.

That said, the Holy Spirit isn't a genie who gives us permission to poof away our enemies into thin air, or who allows us to heal others at whim. He is a person who expresses God's love and power through us, but according to His will, not ours. So amazing is His love within us that He even enables us to pray for those who despise us and love those who are least deserving of our kindness.

Not only does God empower us to live above sin and be healed of our emotional wounds, but according to Isaiah's prophecy, He also heals our physical wounds, because of Jesus' work on the Cross. This is evidenced by the words, "Himself took our infirmities and bare our sicknesses." Meaning, Jesus bore our diseases in His physical body as He hung on the Cross, so that we would not have to bear them ourselves.

So because of Jesus' sacrifice, we have power not only over sin, but also sickness. Anyway, if the Spirit cooperates with the human mind for emotional healing, then why would the Spirit heal the emotions and mind (brain) but leave the rest of the body behind? People with chronic illness generally suffer from symptoms in both mind and body, and healing in the spirit necessarily brings about healing to these areas, too, but we must understand the magnitude of the gift that we have been given in order to appropriate it. We must know that the Spirit of the living God can dwell inside of us and that He has the power to accomplish all things, including the total health of our bodies.

The Spirit Is More Effective In a Sound Mind and Body

Disease in the mind negatively affects our relationship with God and may hinder His ability to operate fully within us. So if a diseased mind limits the work of the Spirit, then wouldn't God desire for the brain and the rest of the body to be healed, also? If you doubt that disease in the mind negatively affects our relationship with God and His ability to work through us, I invite you to read Chapter Eight, where I discuss how dysfunctional biochemistry in the brain affects belief, thoughts, cognition and memory and ultimately, how we view God and the world. Yes, God's Spirit is above all things and can overcome and heal the biochemistry and all that exists in the physical world. Nobody's mind is perfect, but to the degree that the mind is well, and we are submitted to God, the Spirit can operate more fully. So if "by his bruise we are healed", and especially if our sickness is a result of trauma or emotional distress, then healing the mind and body is important if we are to walk in complete spiritual health and carry out God's works of love on earth.

In the Bible, Jesus Healed Everyone!

The New Testament gospels, which describe Jesus' miracles and ministry, provide further evidence of God's willingness to heal. During his ministry on earth, Jesus healed everyone who crossed his path and sensed their need of Him. Whenever he forgave, he also healed. Nobody got left out. Healing was a significant part of His ministry. Why shouldn't it be the same today? It's not as if in modern times God said, "Oh well, never mind, let's not heal their bodies anymore, even though that's been our usual practice over the past ten thousand years. But we'll still forgive their sins." If Jesus Christ "is the same yesterday, today and forever," (Hebrews 13:8) then we can expect to receive the same mercies and gifts of compassion today that He gave His people yesterday. Besides, if it was His compassion that moved Him to heal the sick yesterday, then wouldn't He have that same compassion upon His people today? We have medicine, but medicine doesn't heal many of the chronically ill and not everyone has access to medicine.

Also, there are more diseases on earth today than in Biblical times. Surely God has something better for those left out in the cold! Surely He doesn't mean to leave the gift of healing to only the rich and privileged who can afford the best medical care.

So if He is as compassionate today as yesterday, and the same Spirit that enabled Him to work miracles in Biblical times still operates in people today, then He must be willing to heal those who call upon Him today, too. As a friend once said to me, "If Jesus walked the earth today do you think that he would heal you?" Of course! Jesus no longer walks the earth as a man, but he is still Lord over mankind and Creation.

The following Bible verses exemplify His willingness to heal everyone who approached Him in his day:

Matthew 9:35-36; 10:1. "Then Jesus went about all the cities and villages, teaching in their synagogues, and proclaiming the good news of the kingdom, and curing *every disease and every sickness*. When he saw the crowds, he had compassion for them, because they were harassed and helpless, like sheep without a shepherd ...Then Jesus summoned his twelve disciples, and gave them authority over unclean spirits, to cast them out, and to cure *every disease and every sickness.*"

Matthew 4: 23-25. "Jesus went throughout Galilee, teaching in their synagogues and proclaiming the good news of the kingdom and curing *every sickness and every disease* among the people. So his fame spread throughout all Syria: and they brought to him all the sick, those who were afflicted with various diseases and pains, demoniacs, epileptics and paralytics, and he cured them."

Matthew 12:15. "When Jesus became aware of this (that the Pharisees wanted to destroy him), he departed. Many crowds followed him, and *he cured all of them.*"

The "all's" and "every's" continue throughout the book of Matthew when referring to those whom Jesus healed. Matthew 14:14 and Matthew 14:34-36 provide two more examples, and the books of Luke, Mark and John provide others.

Jesus often required faith from those who wanted to be healed. In the books of Matthew and Luke, a centurion came to Jesus to request that Jesus heal his servant. He said to Jesus, "...but only speak the word and my servant will be healed." Jesus' response to the centurion was, "Go; let it be done for you according to your faith.' And the servant was healed in that hour." Another instance where Jesus cites faith as being important for receiving healing is found in Matthew 9:22 (also mentioned in the books of Mark, Chapter 5, verses 21-43 and Luke 8:40-56). A woman who had been losing blood for years thought to herself, "If I only touch his (Jesus') cloak, I will be made well." After she was healed, Jesus' response to her was, "Take heart, daughter; your faith has made you well." In Matthew 9:28, two blind men came to Jesus for healing. Jesus asked them, "Do you believe that I am able to do this?" To which the blind men replied, "Yes, Lord.' Then Jesus touched their eyes, and said, "According to your faith let it be done to you."

I have known God to heal people who didn't believe in Him, but in general, faith matters. We shouldn't fret over the quality of our faith. Instead, we should keep our eyes focused upon Jesus' work and promises, because this is what heals us.

His Word Has the Power to Heal

The words of the Bible (which are collectively referred to as "the Word") have divine power to create and destroy, and to alter and make manifest in the physical world what doesn't yet exist. Hebrews 11:3 states that, "Through faith we understand that the worlds were prepared by the word of God, so that what is seen was made from things that are not visible." That is, Creation came into existence by the Word. God literally spoke the world into being, and today, by the power and direction of the Holy Spirit, we can also bring into existence things that are not yet, and destroy things that are, by speaking His Word. It's an amazing power and ability that He has given us by His Spirit, but which few take hold of. This is why prayer is so powerful. Prayer can literally move mountains when what is being prayed is according to God's will and timing. Yet, even those of us who claim to believe that there is supernatural power released when we speak God's Word don't always believe it. If we did, we would be meditating more upon its verses and affirming God's promises. For years, I used to listen to preachers proclaim, "There is power in the Word", but I didn't assimilate this truth into my spirit since I read and studied the Bible but seldom witnessed its words altering my life. Occasionally, I would write verses on note cards and study them, but my unbelief kept me from experiencing their power. So I assumed that reading and speaking the word was akin to practicing positive affirmations, and like many others, I maintained my Bible-reading habit, but chucked the idea of meditating upon, and speaking, the Word. It just didn't do much for me, because I didn't yet trust God and didn't have much of a relationship with Him.

After about five years of following Him, He finally convinced me that I was living a less-than victorious existence by not meditating upon its verses and digesting them as if they were as integral to my existence as my daily bread. When this realization began to seep into my soul, I became motivated once again to study the Word and incorporate it into my thoughts. Nearly three years later, I'm still learning to make it a part of my daily thoughts, speech and conduct but now, on the days when I'm able to do this, I notice a difference in how I feel and think. I experience much more peace, wisdom and strength throughout the day. Sometimes, I also feel physically better as a result.

Because God's Word is above circumstances and all created things, speaking and meditating upon His healing promises can dismantle disease in the body and tear down strongholds of darkness in the mind. So we must stand firm upon its promises, trust and believe that these will be eventually fulfilled. In Isaiah 55:11, God says: "...so shall my word be that goes out from my mouth; it shall not return to me empty, but it shall accomplish that which I purpose, and succeed in the thing for which I sent it." Whenever the verses that we speak have the breath of the Holy Spirit upon them, we can be certain that the promises contained within those verses will be accomplished. As we witness their fulfillment, we realize that we are, "calling into existence the things that do not exist" (Romans 4:17) just as God has done since the creation of the universe!

How many thousands of dollars and hours we will spend on treatments and doctors, but how few we will dedicate to prayer and proclaiming the promises of the Bible! Is it because deep down, we think that God won't come through for us? Have we become too accustomed to speaking words of defeat and declaring symptoms? Does the task of changing our words feel too daunting? Do we believe that we are slaves to our minds, that we aren't worthy of health or that God's promises of healing are only for a select few? Such questions reflect the lies that we have been programmed to believe, but which God will help us to overcome if we are willing.

It may be difficult to remember to meditate upon and speak God's truths. But if we know that the words of the Bible are truth and we want to be healed badly enough, then why won't we find ways to incorporate those truths into our hearts?

I believe that God speaks to us in our thoughts and one day, I got the impression that He wanted me to tape Scripture verses all over my apartment, because seeing the verses everywhere would remind me to meditate upon them. For awhile, they did, and as I studied and spoke them, day after day, I discovered that the Word was changing me. The verses didn't sink into my soul and impact my thoughts, feelings or circumstances right away. But when I consistently studied them and spoke them aloud, over time, I experienced little victories in my life and thinking.

Many people pray, go to church and read the Bible, but few use Scripture as a weapon to dismantle disease, dark thoughts and all that is wrong with their lives. We have an adversary in this world; an evil spirit named Satan (or the devil), who doesn't want us to know of the Bible's great power and who will use any means possible to distract, discourage and detour us from accessing it. Because the Bible is one of the greatest sources of power and wisdom on earth, and it demonstrates God's great love for humanity, the truths contained within it are what Satan would most want to keep out of our understanding. This is why, when many people read the Bible, they are confused, disbelieve it, feel condemned, or simply misjudge the intent behind its words and end up thinking that God is violent and angry. Especially if they never read the whole thing! The enemy of our souls prevents us from seeing it for what it really is, and from taking hold of the healing contained within its pages. Those that desire to know the truth, however, will find it, and discover the most powerful weapon on earth. Sometimes, it takes time. Strongholds are called strongholds for a reason, but we can tear these down by the power of the Spirit that dwells within us.

Disease Is Never Called a Blessing in the Bible

Even though God may allow sickness for a season because it conse-crates and sanctifies us, nowhere in the Bible does God call disease a blessing. The sanctification is a blessing, but the disease itself is a curse. In the Old Testament, God sometimes allowed, or even caused, disease to fall upon His people in order to discipline them, but it was always with the ultimate goal of healing them and/or bringing them back into loving relationship with Him. But today, we are under a different covenant—one of everlasting grace. Because of Jesus Christ's work on the Cross, God no longer punishes people for their sins. God may use disease to consecrate us to Him, but He is never its author and whenever He allows it, it's ultimately with the goal of healing us completely, inside and out. He's not angry and He doesn't use disease to punish us. He hates disease and calls it a curse, and promises to heal us from that curse, if we will trust Him and allow Him to do it His way and in His timing.

His Name Is Jehovah-Rapha: "I Am the Lord That Heals Thee"

Jehovah is God's name in the Old Testament when referring to His capacity to redeem, and in the Old Testament books, Jehovah has seven compound names, each one pertaining to a specific redemptive gift that God has given us because of Christ's work on the Cross, and which is intended to meet all of our needs. Those names are:

Jehovah-Shammah, which means "The Lord Is There", and reveals to us our redemptive privilege of being able to enjoy God's presence and be welcome in it.

Jehovah-Shalom, which means "The Lord Our Peace." We can have peace through a relationship with Him, no matter what trials life throws at us.

Jehovah-Ra-ah, which means, "The Lord My Shepherd". He watches over, guides and protects us, as a shepherd would his sheep. On the Cross, Jesus gave His life for His sheep (His followers), so this name also refers to the gift of redemption which God gave us by sending Jesus to be an atoning sacrifice for our sins.

Jehovah-Jireh, which means "The Lord Will Provide." God promises to meet all of our needs; physical, material, spiritual and otherwise. This name also refers to Christ being the offering that God provided for our complete redemption from death and our sinful nature.

Jehovah-Nissi, which means, "The Lord Is Our Banner" (or Victor, or Captain). He has given us victory over death through His work on the Cross, as well as over the darkness and all that conspires to take us into the pit of despair and destruction here on earth. Because the Lord is our Victor, He fights for us and enables us to triumph through difficult circumstances.

Jehovah-Tsidkenu, which means, "The Lord Our Righteousness." Through Jesus' work on the Cross, we are made righteous, or given right standing with Him. Because He became an atoning sacrifice for our sins, we no longer have to try to be good enough for Him. We no longer have to feel guilt and shame for our mistakes. We are perfect in his sight and greatly loved by Him.

…and finally, Jehovah-Rapha, which means, "I Am the Lord, Thy Physician" or "I Am the Lord That Heals Thee." He is our physician who heals us; in body, mind, soul and spirit.

Most Christians agree that God continues to be all of the above for His people today, but in His office as healer, many argue that He only heals the spirit, and only sometimes, or never, the body. But does a physician heal only the spirit? Why wouldn't this redemptive name refer to healing in the body, too? If He doesn't heal us in our bodies today, then this redemptive name is no longer relevant to who He is today and what He wants to be for us. We then have to question whether any of His promises, as revealed through His redemptive names, still apply to us today.

But how could they not? It would be ridiculous if God continued to be our presence, peace, provider, victor, shepherd, and righteousness— but not our healer. And if millions of His followers are struggling through life at half-throttle, their bodies and brains a mess, despite years of medical treatment, then are they really being healed?

He Promises Healing in Matthew 8: 16-17

Matthew 8:16-17 states: "That evening they brought to him many who were possessed with demons; and he cast out the spirits with a word, and cured all who were sick. This was to fulfill what had been spoken through the prophet Isaiah, "He took our infirmities and bore our diseases."

Critics of supernatural healing contend that Isaiah's prophecy was completely fulfilled during Jesus' time on earth, since Jesus' statement in the book of Matthew seems to indicate this. If this is true, then Isaiah's prophecy has no relevancy for today and can't refer to Jesus taking our sicknesses upon Himself on the Cross, as part of His atoning sacrifice for our sins.

The difficulty with the critics' interpretation is that it doesn't fit the context of the rest of verse 4 and verse 5, because the latter part of verse 4 refers to His suffering on the Cross and how, because of this, we regarded Him as struck down and afflicted by God. Critics don't question verse 5, which refers to our redemption from sin because of His death on the Cross. So if, in the verses immediately following "Surely he has borne our infirmities and carried our diseases", Isaiah writes, "But he was wounded for our transgressions, crushed for our iniquities; upon him was the punishment that made us whole, and by his bruise we are healed"—that is, if by his work on the Cross, he is wounded and bruised to bear our iniquities and free us from sin, once and for all and for all time, then why would the preceding verse also not refer to what he has redeemed us from—for all time? Why would part of verse 4 refer only to Jesus' ministry of physical healing on earth, but the rest of verse 4, as well as verse 5, to Him taking our sins upon himself on the Cross? It would be like putting two completely opposite ideas within the same two verses, which is unlikely.

So the promise of Matthew 8:16-17 not only refers to Jesus' ministry on earth, but also to His redemptive promise of freedom from sickness by His work on the Cross.

Jesus Said, "Greater Works than These You Shall Do"

In John 14:12, Jesus says, "Very truly, I tell you, the one who believes in me will also do the works that I do and, in fact, will do greater works than these, because I am going to the Father. I will do whatever you ask in my name, so that the Father may be glorified in the Son. If in my name you ask me for anything, I will do it."

The works that Jesus is referring to here are all those that the Holy Spirit performs in God's people, from speaking words of love and wisdom, to forgiving the sins of others and healing those in need, so that God's work would continue to be carried out by His Spirit after Jesus departed from the earth. If Jesus could heal and raise people from the dead, then surely the "greater works" we perform through the Spirit are inclusive of these things! The works we do are greater than Jesus', not in quality but in quantity. God's Spirit is now present in people all over the world, which means that His Spirit can affect a greater number of people.

Disease Blocks Us from Being Able to Do God's Work

Most Christians would agree that our main purpose on earth is to love God and share His love with others, and people of other faiths and belief systems generally agree that loving others should be humanity's number one priority. But if we're so sick that we can scarcely stumble out the front door, or manage little more than the occasional run to the grocery store, then how can we be used by God to minister effectively to others? Or if we're so depressed and brain-fogged that we can only think of ourselves and how we're going to push through the day, then how can we love others as we love ourselves? How can we be so noble? When in the throes of a devastating disease, considering and attending to the needs of others is difficult, if not impossible (especially in the case of severe mental and physical illness), when our bodies are clamoring for our full attention. God uses some to minister and serve others while sick (I am an example of that, as I have written two books on Lyme disease and counseled others while suffering from severe symptoms) but what if you're a single mother who is too sick to care for her child? Would it be God's will for that child to grow up in a foster home or with her alcoholic father? What if you have an elderly mother who depends on you to take care of her, but you can't even take care of yourself? Would God want that parent to survive on the streets, "for their own good?" What if you are too sick to use the gifts that God has given you for the good of others? I am fortunate because one of my gifts is communication, and it's a gift that I can use despite my disability because I can work from home on my computer. Not everybody is as functional as I am, though, and not everybody has the ability or opportunity to help others from home. On the other hand, I believe that I would be able to help three times as many people if I were completely well. While we can sometimes love and help others while sick, in most cases, we can accomplish far greater things in health, especially if our mental and emotional health have been affected by disease. Our usefulness to God doesn't depend upon our ability to be productive, but we were given brains, arms, legs and bodies that move for a reason. To go, do, speak, pray, love and many other things.

If God's greatest purpose for us on earth is to love and serve others, then how can we effectively do this if the majority of our life's hours are spent in doing and pursuing treatments just to stay functional? Is searching for the next vitamin or herb, spending hours doing daily detoxification protocol and visiting various doctors and therapists, year after year, God's will? For how many years are we supposed to pursue healing, before we say, "enough is enough?" I can't speak for people who have other illnesses, but for those with chronic Lyme disease, healing can be a full-time job—for years, requiring all the resources of the body, mind and spirit. I used to think that it wasn't normal or healthy for me to dedicate half of my existence to getting better, but, five years, two books and hundreds of conversations later, I now realize that most people with chronic Lyme disease fall into this trap because the disease is so incredibly complicated to treat. And, most often, the treatments must be done for years. Not months, but years, and sometimes, indefinitely. Even the chronically ill who actively participate in society often have energy to do little more than work a part-time or full-time job in order to provide for themselves. They collapse at the end of the day, and sleep away the remainder of their life's hours. They have little or nothing left to give others, because they are too mentally, emotionally and physically drained.

If this is you, I can relate to your suffering! So while God may allow disease for a time, if it's within His power to give us "life abundant" (John 10:10), I don't believe that He would want us stuck on a treatment treadmill for a lifetime. We are on this earth for a reason, and it isn't to spend every hour of every day battling our bodies. God has better plans for us and brighter days ahead, if we believe Him and know that this isn't the life that He means for us to lead. He wants to heal us so that we can share His love with others with smiles on our faces instead of sadness in our countenances.

God's Greater Glory Is Made Manifest When We Are Healed

Andrew Murray, one of history's greatest Christian ministers, argues in his book, *Divine Healing,* that while disease can bring people into greater intimacy with God, this closeness happens only by constraint; that is, the sick become close to Him because they are forced to, not because they would otherwise choose a relationship with Him. He writes: "The sufferer who is led by his sufferings to give glory to God, does it, so to speak, by constraint. If he had health and the liberty to choose, it is quite possible that his heart would turn back to the world."

He contends that greater glory is given to God when people are healed supernaturally than when they are left sick, because when they receive a miracle, they experience His touch upon their lives in such a profound way that after they are made well, they want nothing more than to consecrate their lives to Him. This may not be true of those who are close to God only because illness obliges them to be. Murray expresses this belief through the following quote: "When the Lord heals the body, it is so that He may take possession of it and make it a temple that He (the Holy Spirit) may dwell in. The joy which then fills the soul is indescribable. It is not only the joy of being healed, it is joy mingled with humility and a holy enthusiasm which realizes the touch of the Lord, receiving a new life from Him. In the exuberance of his joy, the healed one exalts the Lord, he glorifies Him by word and deed, and all his life is consecrated to God."

So while God may receive glory in our sicknesses, it may be that greater glory is given to Him when we experience, and others witness, His transformative miracles.

Health Is Part of the Promise of Salvation

In the Bible, the Greek word for salvation is *soteria,* the definition of which implies deliverance, preservation, health, healing and soundness. In the New Testament, it's sometimes used to refer to physical health, and at other times, to the health of the soul. The definition of the word is broad, to show us, in a nutshell, all that we are promised when we receive Jesus Christ's gift of salvation. This gift includes both physical and spiritual healing, since it's used throughout the New Testament to refer to both types. So when we accept His gift of salvation, we get much more than just eternal life; we get healing and His presence with us!

Jesus Commands Us to Heal the Sick

In Mark 16:15-18, Jesus says to his disciples: "Go into all the world, and proclaim the good news to the whole creation. The one who believes and is baptized will be saved; but the one that does not believe will be condemned. And these signs will accompany those who believe; by using my name they will cast out demons; they will speak in new tongues; they will pick up snakes in their hands, and if they drink any deadly thing, it will not hurt them; they will lay their hands on the sick, and they will recover."

Most Christians believe that it's important to follow Jesus' command to proclaim the "good news", yet it's funny how some disregard the rest of what Jesus said in these verses, as if the part about our speaking in new tongues and healing the sick isn't relevant to our lives today. But upon what basis do we make this decision? Why do we split Jesus' words in half and accept the half that suits our worldview and circumstances, and toss away the other? Some theologians argue that healing miracles were done only in Jesus' day as a demonstration of

God's love and power, and to prove that Jesus was the Son of God. But people are looking for a Jesus who is just as alive and real today as He was yesterday; a Jesus who operates in our lives in the same way today that he did over two thousand years ago. They aren't looking for a theology; they want the experience of a real person. Jesus performed healing miracles as a demonstration of his mercy and compassion towards others, and while we can read about this mercy and love in the Bible, it touches us more profoundly when the same Jesus that healed the blind man reaches out and touches us, too. He ceases to be our history lesson and instead becomes our reality. May His kingdom come and His will be done!

Chapter 4

A Few Reasons Why Christians Don't Believe In Miracles

Many Christians believe that God no longer performs healing miracles, because of their personal experiences or faulty church doctrine that they have been taught. Or they believe that miracles aren't common, and consequently, that they aren't one of God's preferred ways of revealing His love. Whether they have lost loved ones to disease or been taught that God no longer heals, the end result is the same: they disbelieve or struggle to believe in a God of miracles. In this chapter, I cite three of the most common arguments that some Christians use to disprove that God heals supernaturally, and then provide counter-arguments to demonstrate that these arguments are based on faulty logic. In doing so, I hope to provide a new, more encouraging perspective for those who struggle to believe in miracles because of what they have seen, experienced or been taught.

Miracles are Rare, and Many Who Pray Don't Get One

Those who don't believe in supernatural healing argue that if God is so keen on miracles, then more of us should have witnessed one by now. If this were a favorite method of God for making people well, then surely, our eyes should have been dazzled by a faith healing at least once! The fact is, most of us have never seen a miracle. Besides, millions of people who beg God for healing remain ill or die in their diseases, no matter how many pleas they offer up to the Heavenlies. Why must they receive a miracle only by someone anointed with the Holy Spirit and the gift of healing? What about the Spirit that dwells within themselves? Why won't that Spirit rise up and heal them, if God does so many miracles?

Well, first, faith can be measured by the level of trust that we have in our relationship with God, and if the unhealed don't trust Him or believe that He wants to heal them, they may be unable to receive His promises.

Second, God is merciful, but the universe is governed by certain spiritual laws. If it's the Holy Spirit that heals, and obtaining healing is dependent upon our ability to receive the Spirit and upon allowing His power to flow through us, then those who don't understand or know this may not be made well.

Is this fair? How about to the millions of people in Africa and Asia who die of AIDS, malaria and malnutrition, and who have never heard the name Jesus Christ, but who pray for healing anyway? What about the millions in Latin America who believe in God's promises of healing, and who pray and plead for years, yet remain sick? What about the mother whose child has cancer but who is unaware that God heals by the power of the Holy Spirit?

Well, whether it's fair or not from our perspective, spiritual laws govern the universe, and in the beginning, God decided that the Holy Spirit indwelling His followers would be His preferred source and method for healing. So prayer for healing may be insufficient if the Holy Spirit isn't present or allowed to operate in a person. Also, if we don't realize the great power that God has given us over disease through Christ's work on the Cross (as discussed in Chapter Three), or if we don't fully believe in Him and His willingness to restore us, then we may not be able to receive from Him.

At the same time, if we cry out for truth, if we implore God for His presence, He will come to us, no matter our country, culture or faith. Evidence for this is found in Jeremiah 29:13 where He says: "When you search for me, you will find me; if you seek Me with all your heart, I will let you find me." So those who desire Him with a pure, hungry and humble heart can and will find Him, and in turn, receive healing by His Spirit.

Miracles aren't as rare as some suppose, though. In churches and nations where the Holy Spirit is allowed to operate, miracles abound. I discovered this truth when I started attending healing conferences and churches where healing was practiced. If we haven't seen a miracle, it may be because we haven't been hanging out in the right places!

Finally, ministers who have been used by God to heal multitudes contend that sin and unforgiveness, as well as other personal "road-blocks", can keep people from receiving healing. So there are sometimes (though not always) conditions to receiving God's healing touch. I discuss this concept more in-depth in the following chapters.

Many Who Believed God for Healing Died Anyway

Some people who believed against all odds that God would heal them have ended up dying in their diseases. Logically, the friends and family members of such faith-filled people disbelieve or struggle to believe that God desires to heal all who seek Him for this gift. After all, why would He allow their loved ones with that much faith to die in their diseases, if His will was for them to be well?

Before we can adopt this as a valid excuse for why God doesn't heal our physical bodies, we must jump into the hearts of those who believed God for a miracle and yet died. Maybe they were harboring unforgiveness against someone, and God was unable to heal them because they chose to not release that forgiveness. Maybe their faith was based upon desperation for a solution, rather than true belief in a loving God who heals. Maybe yet, God had a sovereign reason for allowing them to die, which nobody can or will understand this side of Heaven.

This latter explanation would appear to contradict His promises in the Bible, but life is filled with examples of situations that, on the surface, appear to contradict His Word. In the end, we must decide whether to believe for a miracle based on our experience or on what God has said in the Bible. Is truth what we experience, or is it what God has promised?

The fact that some people die in their diseases, despite God's promises, doesn't negate the truth of His Word and the fact that many others *are* healed by His hand. Convincing proofs of this healing exist in abundance in churches where healing is practiced.

If your confidence has been cast away as a result of having lost loved ones to disease, I understand how difficult it must be to adopt a different perspective on healing. Nonetheless, I encourage you to study Jesus' words and works in the Bible, attend a few healing conferences, and read a handful of books on healing, to see if these help you to re-evaluate the criteria upon which you have based your belief. To embrace a different theology may be too painful, but what if it ends up saving you from a life of illness? To be able to say, "I don't know why my mother passed away, even though her faith in miracles was rock-solid, but I'm going to believe that God wants to heal me anyway," is a bold step of confidence in Jesus' work on the Cross and in God's promises of healing.

The Apostle Paul Had A "Thorn In The Flesh"—A Disease!

According to the Bible, Satan afflicted history's most important evangelist and apostle, Paul, with a "thorn in the flesh." The verse that describes the thorn is found in 2 Corinthians 12:7-10, and states: "Therefore, to keep me from being too elated, a thorn was given me in the flesh, a messenger of Satan to torment me, to keep me from being too elated. Three times I appealed to the Lord about this, that it would leave me, but he said to me, "My grace is sufficient for you, for power is made perfect in weakness. So I will boast all the more gladly of my weaknesses, insults, hardships, persecutions and calamities for the sake of Christ; for whenever I am weak, then I am strong."

The Christian church debates the meaning of Paul's thorn. Critics of supernatural healing tend to argue that the thorn was a disease, and love to cite this verse as evidence for why God doesn't perform miracles today. They argue that if the faith of history's greatest apostle was insufficient to heal him, then why should any of us today expect healing?

Surprisingly, this verse carries more weight in the church on the subject of healing than the multitude of other verses throughout the Bible which promise healing to God's people.

According to F.F. Bosworth, author of *Christ the Healer,* nowhere in the Bible is the expression "thorn in the flesh" used to describe disease. Rather, it is always used to describe an annoying personality, or oppressive spirit. Its use in the Bible is similar to how we use it in speech today. In his book, Bosworth contends that the literal translation for "messenger of Satan" is "angelos" or "angel" of Satan, and of the 188 times that the "angelos" is mentioned in the Bible, in all instances, it refers to a satanic personality, sent by Satan to torment somebody. So a satanic angel was sent to Paul to annoy him. He wasn't struck by disease, according to Bosworth.

Also, some versions of the Bible translate "weaknesses, insults, hardships and persecutions" as "infirmities" (which implies that Paul suffered from disease), but this latter interpretation is based upon earlier translations of the Bible. More ancient manuscripts have since been discovered which have proven this interpretation to be flawed. So the "thorn in the flesh" argument may be overrated, if not flawed.

Even if the "thorn in the flesh" did represent an illness, as some theologians contend, God had allowed it to keep Paul humble, because He had given him an abundance of revelations and didn't want him to become "too elated." I doubt that any of us today are sick because we have received revelations that are as amazing as those of the church's greatest apostle, and that we all need to be humbled because of what we know. Most of us aren't afflicted because we are exceedingly holy, but rather, because we have been badly wounded by life. Many of the chronically ill that I know are humble, holy people, but their illnesses are usually a result of unresolved emotional trauma, an accident, a bug that infected them, or some combination of the three. It would be cruel to believe that God needs to further humble those who have been afflicted by a lifetime of emotional and/or physical trauma by allowing them to be ill.

The Body Is In a Continual State of Decay

Finally, critics of supernatural healing sometimes contend that the body is in a continual state of decay, so if God promises us healing, then we shouldn't sag, bag or get cavities. They believe that after a healing miracle, the body should be made perfect, and if it isn't, then God's promises of healing aren't for real. They think that we should have no need for eyeglasses, silver fillings and Ibuprofen after God touches us, and our cells should become perfect, like those of a child that hasn't been subjected to a toxic environment or fifty years of life.

Because I have seen healing miracles and received them myself, I know that God heals, but He may not restore every cell in the body. Yet, He can and does free us from our burdensome symptoms and restore our ability to lead normal, productive lives. Thus, a person with cancer can be freed of all cancer cells without the remaining cells in the body being made entirely new. A person with hepatitis can have his or her liver repaired without the other organs being restored to perfect functionality. God's healing may mean making all things new in the body, but more often, it means removing the symptoms that hinder us from living productive, happy, functional lives. His goal is to take us out of our misery because He loves us! Just because He doesn't restore every cell in the body doesn't mean that He doesn't remove our infirmities. So in reality, this argument of the critics is no argument at all.

Chapter 5

Factors That Influence Healing and Why Some Don't Receive a Miracle

So what about people who believe God for a miracle but don't get one? As someone who believes in miracles but still has symptoms, I empathize with the scores of chronically ill who have believed and not received, or who have been rebuked by well-meaning Christians who admonished them to "just have more faith". Perhaps they have been told that they are sick because they have unconfessed sin in their lives. The Bible gives numerous examples of how people weren't healed from their illnesses because of unforgiveness and because they departed from God's ways, but the book of Job should refute any argument that personal sin is always the reason for illness. Job was the godliest man of his day, and God allowed him to suffer disease for a time, to test his faith and prove Satan's defeat, but He didn't allow Him to be sick forever.

Nonetheless, it may be helpful for us to ask God the reason for our suffering, because He may want us to understand or do something before He can heal us—with the help of His Spirit, of course! We may receive silence for an answer, or He may give us pearls that will help us find our way to health. Francis McNutt's book, *Healing,* Henry Wright's *A More Excellent Way* and other healing books cite an abundance of reasons why people get blocked in their ability to receive healing from God, and also provide valuable insights into what God sometimes requires of them if they want to be made well. These are based on Biblical truths. For instance, in John 5:6, Jesus asked a man at the pool of Bethesda whether he wanted to be well. He may need for us to ask ourselves the same question and remove the roadblocks that keep us from responding with a resounding "yes!" before He can heal us.

Admittedly, reading over the lists of roadblocks cited in these books, that mention everything from unforgiveness to a lack of belief or inability to surrender to God; focusing on symptoms instead of God's promises, failing to persevere, confessing doubts, and living a sinful life, used to leave me discouraged. I used to think that any person with perfectionist tendencies, like me, and who read such lists, would believe that they could never meet all of the requirements for a miracle. I mean, of course I focus on my symptoms! I spend three to four hours a day doing treatments and taking pills, and my symptoms remind me every two seconds about how broken I am. It can be a superhuman feat for me to not focus on disease. Yes, the Spirit helps us in our weaknesses (Romans 8:26), but the empowerment that we receive from Him also depends in part upon our humility before Him and the degree to which we are able to surrender to Him.

Everyone lives an imperfect and sinful life. We may walk in the path of His Spirit but we still make mistakes. Fortunately, I've learned that it's not up to us to make sure that we're doing everything right. Only God can do that, and empower us to do whatever we need to do to be healed, including teaching us how to surrender and walk in humility before Him.

In their efforts to lead a holy life, some people keep a mental list of well-defined acts and attitudes that are considered to be sinful and which they consequently avoid, such as alcoholism, sexual immorality, and hating one's brother. They conclude that if they aren't committing any of these "major sins", then they aren't living in sin and that God should heal them. But what about those sins seldom talked about in the church, such as attitudes of judgment and self-righteousness? What about pride or feelings of shame towards oneself? What about forgetting to change the toilet roll as a subconscious act of self-sabotage? How about ignoring God when He tells them through a heart tug to pray for someone on the street, or turning a deaf ear to the cries of children in Latin America who need more help from wealthier nations? How do you define what it means to live in sin? I define it by anything that doesn't line up with God's way of doing things, but none of us lives God's way 100% of the time.

So reviewing the list of potential roadblocks to healing can be stifling and imprisoning, if you are a type-A personality like me and tend to forget that you can't earn your healing! Besides, if I scrutinized myself, right down to the last stitch in my soul, I know that all of those healing roadblocks would apply to me. And if they do, then I have to ask myself some torturous, type-A questions, such as: Is God withholding my healing because I still have angry thoughts about so-and-so from time to time? Would I receive a miracle if I focused on my symptoms only twenty percent of the time, instead of fifty? Would God spill Holy Ghost healing confetti over me if I managed to speak words of life instead of death a majority of the time? But is that even possible, if my current medication leaves me depressed and negative? Is healing dependent upon me doing everything right? If you tend to fall into a performance-based, type-A mindset over this issue, as I have, you can drive yourself crazy just trying to figure it all out!

At the same time, the laundry lists of roadblocks to healing have validity, because the ministers who have compiled them are witnesses to why people aren't healed. They see miracles happen when, with the help of the Holy Spirit, the sick manage to attend to their roadblocks and remove them from their lives. Also, in the Bible, God *does* cite reasons why people don't get better, everything from a lack of faith to unforgiveness, as well as others. He also mentions factors that sometimes enable healing, such as considering the poor, praying for others, and speaking words of truth. We don't have to be perfect but we must give God something to work with so that we don't block His healing hand with our unforgiveness, unbelief, or whatever sin is keeping us from receiving His touch. For example, an intention to forgive, or a willingness to speak His promises of healing in the morning, can open the door to receiving from Him. When we ask the Spirit to help us in our weaknesses, He will reveal to us the things that are blocking us and enable us to take hold of that which God so desires to give us.

So don't let the checklist overwhelm you. Instead, consider the factors that block, as well as enable healing, and ask God to reveal whether any of them apply to you. You will know the answer because you will feel a tug in your spirit if they do. Then ask Him to guide you in your thoughts and actions, so that you can more fully cooperate with Him in your healing process. Don't do what I used to do and analyze the matter to death. If you constantly wonder how you've kept God's hands tied, you're walking in performance –based faith, which isn't what He wants. He gives us all things to His children by grace, and by the empowerment of His Spirit. If we ask Him, He will show and enable us to do, or receive, all that we need from Him. So in the end, it's really about His efforts, along with our willingness to trust and yield to Him.

Also, according to the Bible, how we live affects our ability to receive healing from God, but not always because God requires us to do something before we can receive from Him. When we live and act upon His Word, our hearts and spirits are moved in such a manner that enables us to receive and live in His love. As a byproduct of living in His love, we get healed.

What Enables Healing

Loving Others and Providing for the Poor

The first few lines of Psalm 41:1 read: "Happy are those who consider the poor; the Lord delivers them in the day of trouble. The Lord protects them and keeps them alive; they are called happy in the land. You do not give them up to the will of their enemies. The Lord sustains them on their sickbed; in their illness you heal all their infirmities."

From this verse, we learn that God is compassionate towards those who show compassion for others, and heals those who consider the afflictions of the poor. Also, when we help the poor, we live in God's love, and by itself, that love can heal us, in body, mind and spirit.

Another Bible verse that links healing to helping the poor and loving others in a variety of ways is found in Isaiah 58:6-8: "Is this not the fast that I (the Lord) choose? To loose the bonds of injustice, to undo the thongs of the yoke, to let the oppressed go free, and to break every yoke? Is it not to share your bread with the hungry, and bring the homeless poor into your house; when you see the naked, to cover them, and not to hide yourself from your own kin? Then your light shall break forth like the dawn, and *your healing shall spring up quickly*; your vindicator shall go before you, the glory of the Lord shall be your rear guard."

"Loosing the bands of injustice" in these verses can refer to doing the right thing amidst fierce opposition, and fighting to free those in bondage to unfair laws, harmful relationships and other situations where we observe wrongdoing. "Undoing the thongs of the yoke and letting the oppressed go free" may refer to changing our attitude and actions towards those whom we have harmed through our unforgiveness and selfishness. It may also refer to allowing God to set us free from the oppression and burdens that we subject ourselves to, when we allow sinful thoughts and actions to dominate our lives. When we follow these commands, we become freed from the bondage of the world and the grip that Satan has on our lives. As we are freed, we are healed. A life of bondage and selfishness makes the body sick; a life of love and freedom heals it.

Other verses in the Bible describe how our attitudes and actions affect our health. Psalms and Proverbs are two books that provide a plethora of such verses.

Speaking and Meditating Upon Truth

Speaking and meditating upon Biblical truths can also heal the body, mind and spirit, in a number of ways.

For example, Proverbs 4: 20-22 states: "My child, be attentive to my words; incline your ear to my sayings. Do not let them escape from your sight; keep them within your heart. For they are life to those who find them, and *healing to all their flesh.*"

King Solomon, the wisest king to ever rule Israel, wrote most of the proverbs by divine revelation from God. In these verses, the words and sayings that he is referring to are those which God gave him (us). Meditating upon God's words and sayings heals the body because our cells respond favorably whenever our thoughts reflect His loving attributes of righteousness, wisdom, kindness, compassion and so on. The body is broken by unloving attitudes, as evidenced by other proverbs. I.e.; Proverbs 14:30 says, "A tranquil mind gives life to the flesh, but passion (as in fierce anger) makes the bones rot." Science and medicine have also proven that attitudes of negativity, bitterness, unforgiveness and anger make the body sick.

Similarly, Proverb 16:24 confirms the power of words to heal. "Pleasant words are like a honeycomb, *sweetness to the soul, and health to the body.*"

Speaking words of love and light, even those that aren't contained within Bible verses, also heals us. We often become what we meditate upon, and if most of our thoughts and spoken words are negative then we will struggle to heal. How many of us spend our thoughts and speech on attitudes which result from self-pity, worry, anger and fear!

Bruce Lipton, an anatomy professor who holds a PhD in developmental cell biology, has written an excellent book called *Biology of Belief,* which provides scientific evidence to demonstrate how our thoughts affect our biochemistry. He contends that the body's genes, or DNA, are controlled and influenced by energetic signals from outside the cell. These signals come from our internal, as well as external, environment. He writes that some of these signals, or energetic messages, emanate from our thoughts. So our thoughts affect our DNA and every cell in our bodies!

The body doesn't function solely by biochemical processes; scientific discoveries have proven, and are proving, that its processes happen first and foremost on an energetic level, and subsequently, on a biochemical level. Matter is comprised of energy (remember Einstein's equation?), so according to Lipton, changes in the body's DNA results from changes in its energetic field, and the thoughts influence this energetic field! So Lipton's work provides an excellent example of how some Biblical truths can be explained on a scientific level.

As previously mentioned, speaking Biblical truths also heals us because there is supernatural power behind the Word, which, when spoken, demolishes invisible spiritual strongholds of darkness that oppress us in our minds and bodies.

Our attitude towards God and how we live affects our ability to receive healing from Him, too. Reverencing, trusting and looking to Him for wisdom, instead of relying solely upon our own fleshly (or carnal) thoughts to get us through life, can positively influence health. Proverbs 3:7-8 says: "Do not be wise in your own eyes: fear the Lord, and turn away from evil. It *will be a healing for your flesh and a refreshment for your body.*"

Other verses in the Bible describe additional factors that influence healing, but in a nutshell, our faith and obedience to God are most important, which include meditating upon and speaking His promises. Yet receiving healing isn't about meeting a set of requirements, but rather, creating an atmosphere where healing becomes possible.

Being Willing to Surrender Our Lives to Him

Once, I thought I heard God ask me whether I would consecrate my entire life to Him, if He healed me. Not could I, but would I, if He enabled me? Would I be willing to give up my hateful thoughts towards those who had wounded me in the past? Could I resist rolling in the muck of self-pity and instead take pity upon another, even if they didn't deserve it? Could I squelch the urge to complain about my life and instead thank God for my healing, even though it hadn't yet manifest? Was I fed up enough with feeling horrible to embrace the difficult work of change? He had already healed my mind and spirit of many things, but He wanted me to go deeper. As I pondered such questions, I realized that I had moved from a "stuck" place of believing that I couldn't do these things, to a place of feeling able. Yet my willingness lagged. Did I want to be healed badly enough, in body, mind and spirit?

Finally, one day, I decided that I did, but I had to get really sick of my life and everything in it before I felt empowered enough to change—and only because the alternative was a life of sheer misery. In the end, though, it has been the greatest blessing, as the Holy Spirit has not only empowered me, but brought greater joy and peace into my life because I chose to cooperate with Him and take the higher road. And as I surrender to Him and walk this higher road, I feel increasingly better in my physical body, as well as in my spirit and emotions.

Surrendering to God and walking His path can be challenging, but when we do, it brings healing to our whole person. Because God is love and when we surrender to and obey Him, we walk in that love, and it heals all of our brokenness.

If we ask God, He will show us—through our thoughts, circumstances, people, prayer and other means, all that we need to know in order to be healed. If we don't get an answer, then He may only want us to be patient, trust Him, and peacefully wait for His plan to unfold. And don't worry—He'll help you with the patience, too!

Allowing Him to Heal Us His Way, Not Ours

Over the past year, I have received several prophecies regarding my healing. The first came from a woman named Maria, who attended my Bible study group in Costa Rica. Known among those in the neighborhood for her ability to hear God, she would often get up in the middle of the night to pray. My last night at the Bible study before leaving

Costa Rica, she said to me, "God says that He gave you health on the Cross at Calvary, but you need to believe Him a little more for it." She spoke several other prophecies over me, which revealed truths about me that she couldn't have known had God not told her, and which convinced me that her words were sent from Him. These words gave me hope, because through her, I learned that God wanted me to be well, and that He would lead me towards a better life.

Approximately six months later, a prophetic friend in my church said, "God just told me that He's healing you gradually…to build your faith."

Recently, this same prophetic friend said, "God says, My servant shall be healed….after a short season."

Even more recently, another friend from Costa Rica said, "God says that your healing has already been released from Heaven and will manifest in you soon."

I also received three prophecies this year in which God told me, through three different people, that He wanted me to let go of the need to be healed immediately, and instead trust His timing in the process!

All of these prophecies confirmed a few things for me. First, God had already provided healing to me through Jesus Christ's work on the Cross, but the manifestation of that healing was happening slowly, because He yet needed to build my faith. Secondly, His healing isn't always instantaneous. Sometimes, the miracle happens over time. Thirdly, I needed to trust His timing in the process.

God may take the slow path with us, for some good purpose, such as getting us to renounce our unforgiveness towards others, or so that we will learn to believe in His promises, because belief in His willingness to heal us matters, if we want to receive it.

His ways aren't our ways. Isaiah 59: 9 states: "For as the heavens are higher than the earth, so are my ways higher than your ways and my thoughts than your thoughts." We should expect healing, but in His time and according to His ways.

Taking Communion

Communion is the act of taking bread and fruit of the vine (wine or grape juice) as a reminder of all that Jesus has done for us, and especially, His work on the Cross. The bread represents His body, which has been broken for us, and the wine, or juice, represents His blood, which was shed for the forgiveness of our sins.

Perry Stone, in his book, *The Meal That Heals,* writes that we can receive physical, spiritual and emotional healing from God by taking communion, if we believe in the healing power of Christ's body and blood. This is because the redemptive anointing of Christ works through us to heal us whenever we take communion.

He writes: "Communion is powerful because it's based upon God's covenant with us. When I receive Communion, I sense such a relief knowing that I am leaning, not on another person's prayers or another person's faith, but upon simple trust in God's covenant."

As we take communion, we can meditate upon the fact that when Jesus died, He not only forgave us of our sins, but as Isaiah 53 mentions, also took our diseases upon Himself, so that we wouldn't have to suffer them. Taking the bread and wine is an affirmation that we have been forgiven and made a "new creation in Christ" (2 Cor. 5:17), since His death and resurrection made it possible for the Holy Spirit to indwell us, heal us and give us new life. In John 16:7, Jesus says to His disciples, "...it is to your advantage that I go away, for if I do not go away, the Advocate (Holy Spirit) will not come to you; but if I go, I will send Him to you".

Meditating upon Jesus' death on the Cross and how this event purchased our redemption from sickness and sin increases our faith for healing. Taking Communion provides an opportunity for us to meditate upon this truth as well as a tangible way for us to embrace it. Provided, of course, we believe that physical healing was part of the gift that He gave us when He sacrificed Himself on our behalf. We must know that we were redeemed from both sin and sickness when He died, and that He paid an immense price for us to be freed from its bondage.

Why We Become Blocked in Our Ability to Receive from God

One of the most common, and important, blocks to healing is a lack of realization of how much God loves us. Yes, God can work miracles, regardless of our opinion of Him and ourselves, but sometimes, we fail to receive because our perception of Him and how He sees us is flawed.

We Don't Know How Much He Loves Us

F.F. Bosworth, on page 74 of *Christ the Healer*, writes, "It is not faith in God's power that secures His blessings but faith in His love and in His will."

So many things in the world conspire against us having faith in His love and will! In the preceding chapters, I mentioned some reasons why I believe that it's God's will for everyone to be well, as well as reasons why some aren't healed. In this one, I discuss how trauma and harmful beliefs, which result from our environment, upbringing, and lack of knowledge of God's love for us, block us in our ability to receive from Him. In this chapter, as well as in Chapter Seven, I suggest some practical solutions for removing these blocks and learning to have faith in His love, so that we can, in turn, believe Him for healing. These solutions are based on what He has taught me over the past eight years in my own healing journey.

Trauma Creates a False Concept of His Love

For many of us, our faith in God's love has been devastated by the hardships we have suffered, especially early in life. By uncles that abused us. By daddies and stepmothers who were tyrants and who gave us our first impressions of humanity. By mothers who denied us our needs, and teachers and peers who made fun of us and treated us un-kindly. If our perceptions of love were defined mostly by people who knew little about its true meaning themselves, we grew up not knowing the difference between right and wrong; between a loving action and an unloving one. Love and hate got confused. Our foundation was built in a faulty way.

Many experts claim that, if unchallenged, our image of God mirrors that which we have of our father figures, or primary caregivers. If Dad was demanding, then God must be, too. If Grandpa was critical, then so is God. If Aunt Nellie was kind, then so is God. While true, the problem with this argument is that it can be used as an excuse for not being able to experience God's love, because it necessarily implies that those who have lived through the greatest tragedies have the least chance of experiencing God's love. This would then mean that a loving God is only for the happy and sane who were lucky enough to have relatively well-balanced parents or caretakers.

Fortunately, God is bigger than our images and imaginations, and while these are influenced by how our primary caregivers treated us, He can reveal Himself to us in powerful ways, so that over time, we learn to see what true love looks like. The Bible is full of whacked-out, dysfunctional people to whom God revealed His love. He delights in demonstrating His love to the most wounded and sinful of souls, and often uses such people to accomplish His highest purposes. This is so that His incredible redemptive power will be made manifest to others. And the darker our lives, the more His transformative light can shine brightly into them, to be seen by others.

I have seen God take some of the saddest, angriest people and make miracles of their lives. Some have been changed instantaneously by a direct, powerful revelation of His love, in the form of a Holy Ghost warm fuzzy or as a profound revelation of what Christ did for them on the Cross. More often, though, I have witnessed them transformed slowly, by years of prayer and time spent with God; through counseling, circumstances, studying the Word and experiencing the love of other godly people.

Unfortunately, studying the Bible doesn't help everyone at the outset of their faith walk. I have friends who, as children, were whacked over the head with the Bible, or constantly criticized and told that God would send them to Hell if they didn't study and obey it. These friends fear the Bible and it reads like a book of condemnation to them. Before I understood the implications of God's grace, parts of the Bible felt condemning to me, too. It's only as God has provided me with an ever-increasing revelation of His love for me that I have been able to read the Bible with eyes of truth and receive it with a heart of love. Now, it's my lifeline and I can't live without it. It transforms, empowers and enriches my existence.

But God's healing promises may mean little to those who have Bible-phobia and consequently, little knowledge of His love for them. Because they can't study the Word and through it, understand that God wants to heal them, they become hindered in their ability to receive His gifts.

If you are one of these people, you may receive healing if the Word is presented to you in a different format, such as through a friend who speaks it to you, in song, prayer or conversation. Asking God to reveal and break the mental strongholds that may prevent you from being able to read and receive its truths is important, too. Keep in mind, not every word in the Bible will be relevant and applicable to your life today, so if the verses don't speak to your heart, they probably aren't meant for you to understand right now. It's okay. You can leave them for a later day.

Subconscious Motivations Keep Us Sick

Some people have subconscious motivations for remaining sick. This blocks them from receiving healing from God, because a part of them really doesn't want to be well. The deep-seated fears that they harbor and which cause them to subconsciously want to stay stuck in their diseases are valid, but need to be identified so that they can resolve them on a conscious level and get healed. Below I describe what some of these motivations are.

→ *Disease Enables Us to Avoid Rejection and Life:* Some people remain ill out of a subconscious desire to escape society. This is often due to a fear of rejection; from those in the workplace, loved ones, and the world at large. Disease provides them with an excuse to not engage in society, so that they don't have to endure the possibility of loss. Such people have usually experienced extreme rejection in their lives from their primary caretakers or loved ones. Resolving the rejection requires first recognizing its role in perpetuating disease, then stepping out and doing what is most uncomfortable; engaging with others.

If this is you, you might argue that you aren't well enough to participate in activities with others. While that may be legitimately true, if you have unresolved rejection fears, it may also be part of your mind's ploy to keep you safe. Resolving these fears with a counselor is helpful, although the roots of rejection can be so deep that only a profound revelation of God's love, given by the Holy Spirit, can obliterate the deep feelings of inadequacy that block healing.

Often, God heals our rejection by teaching us to see ourselves as He sees us. He may, for instance, through a pastor or our prayers, show us that our value and worth aren't determined by how others treat us. When we seek approval from others, we abdicate our value to them. We let them decide by their approval of us what we are worth. God may then show us that this is foolishness, because the only opinion that matters is His, and He thinks that we are worth dying for! Nothing we do can diminish His adoration of us. We are greater than gold and all of the universe's treasures, simply because He made us. He encourages us to believe that only He can provide us with an objective assessment of our worth, because only He is perfect. Because we are flawed and wounded, we aren't qualified to assign worth to another, and neither should we allow our worth to be determined by others' words and actions towards us.

Another way that God may heal our rejection is by showing us that He doesn't blame us for our failures. He knows the traumas that we have suffered. He is aware of every last blow that has ever been dealt to us; every foul word and curse that has ever been spoken against us, and He understands how these have hurt us. He doesn't expect us to walk away from abuse unscathed. He doesn't expect us to forgive and forget in a day. Instead, He holds us in our pain and tells us that He has cried with us in our suffering. He accepts us, and understands how our wounds have caused us to make serious mistakes in our relationships. He sympathizes with our pain. Knowing this can heal our hearts.

God works in other ways to heal rejection (some of which are described later in this book). But we must rise above our fears and believe that He's not going to let us down! We must take a risk, because He who is faithful has promised to redeem us.

→ *Disease Is A Way to Get Sympathy (Love) From Others:* Another subconscious motivation for illness is to get sympathy and attention from others. This is really borne out of a need for love. If we were deprived of love in our early childhood years, or if a spouse or partner aren't loving us as we think they should, then we may become, or remain, sick in order to quietly solicit the sympathy of others and in turn, get our love needs met. If people won't love us in health, the subconscious reasons, maybe they will love us through our infirmities. This reasoning may be particularly applicable if, as a child, our primary caregivers were only kind and loving towards us when we had colds or flus or broken arms. We may have learned that infirmity is the only way to receive love, so we remain ill in order to get this need met. Correspondingly, we may not be able to receive God's gift of physical healing until we receive revelation of His love and realize that sickness is a counterproductive way to get our needs met.

The revelation of that love may come over time, but in the Bible, He promises that we will find Him if we seek Him with all of our heart (Jeremiah 29:13). God is love, and to seek Him is to find genuine, radiant, and healthy love. In the meantime, resisting the urge to complain about our sad lot in life can break our powerful addiction to sympathy. Sometimes we need comfort and to be heard by others, but when the soul constantly begs for attention, it is in bondage. Receiving sympathy from others may temporarily relieve our need for comfort, but like a drug, we may find ourselves clamoring for another hit the next day. And if sickness provides an excuse for us to receive sympathy, we may subconsciously choose to remain ill. Recognizing that sickness is an illusory place for our love needs to get met, and resisting the urge to complain, will free us.

Unquestionably, chronic illness causes immense suffering and we may legitimately need a lot of love and support from others. Having friends and family to whom we can express our pain and suffering is crucial for our healing. It can be difficult to discern the difference between a healthy expression of pain and an addiction to complaining, but if we go to God and ask Him for discernment, He will show us when our "venting" is no longer healthy. When the complaining is constant, and lasts for many months or years, this may be one warning sign that we have become addicted to the need for sympathy-- especially if our conversations with others seem to revolve mostly around our problems and those problems never get solved. We must break these patterns, with the help of God and His ministers, if we want to be free.

→ *We Use Disease to Punish and/or Protect Ourselves:* The need to punish or protect ourselves or others may be another subconscious motivation for illness. For example, if we harbor unforgiveness against ourselves for betraying our spouse or children, we may believe that we need to be punished for that. Or we may think that God wants to punish us for our evil deeds by allowing us to be sick. We must know that God's amazing grace is greater than any foul act that we could ever commit, and accept in our hearts that Jesus died so that we might be released from the shackles of guilt and shame. But if something within us yet believes that we don't deserve to be well, and we keep inwardly lashing ourselves, then we may not receive His healing. If we meditate upon the fact that it isn't holy or pleasing to God when we punish ourselves for our past sins, this can help free us from our guilt. If we ask Him to remind us of the incredible price that He paid to free us from shame, guilt and self-hatred, and to reveal to our hearts the impli-cations of what that means for our lives, we may be able to release the condemnation that binds us to disease. I have found that taking com-munion on a daily or weekly basis reminds me of Jesus' work, as it makes the freedom that He gave me from sin and sickness a more tangible reality in my life.

We may also use disease to punish our loved ones for their crimes against us. If being sick prevents us from being available to them or meeting their needs, or if it forces them to become our full-time care-takers, then it may be a subconscious way that we exact revenge upon them for hurting us. If we have trouble setting boundaries with others, we can fall prey to this type of manipulative behavior. This is because if we can't express our needs and feelings in a constructive manner, then resentment builds, and that resentment must go somewhere. If we don't express it verbally, then our bodies will express it through symptoms, and until we recognize that we are harboring some ugly stuff and deal with it, our healing won't manifest. Learning to express our opinions and needs in a constructive manner, without fearing what others will think of or do to us, is important. We must also forgive ourselves and others, so that we can stop punishing them and ourselves with symptoms. Forgiveness is discussed more in-depth later in this chapter.

→ *Disease Is Too Comfortable:* Chronic illness is a living hell, anything but comfy-cozy, but to a mind and body accustomed to self-sabotage, it may be the safest, cushiest place for the soul to be.

It has often been said that those who have suffered from abuse as children, seek spouses that resemble their abusive caretakers. The patterns of behavior exhibited in abuse are what they are familiar with, and humans crave familiarity. The dysfunctional patterns of behavior in abusive people feel safe to the abused, and because they have learned to believe that this is what they deserve, they shun relationships that offer true love. They would rather suffer infinite pain than face their fear of the unknown—which is healthy love.

Prison inmates, after they are freed, often commit crimes so that they will be put back in jail, because they have become so accustomed to confinement that they can't handle being in the world. Incarceration is what they know, and while living behind bars is no kind of life, the world outside is just too frightening for them.

The same phenomenon can happen with the chronically ill, who have become so accustomed to living in infirmity that they are more comfortable with their pain and isolation from society than they are with the people and things of the world. This happens to the strongest of the strong, because learning to find contentment in confinement is a necessary evil in order to survive the isolation and disability of chronic illness.

During the first months that I suffered from severe symptoms of Lyme disease, I frequently dreamed that I was in prison. From my cell, I would watch the world, active, happy and healthy around me. In desperation, I pleaded for God to let me out of jail; this wasn't the kind of life I had signed up for and I wanted out! Oh, how these dreams devastated my soul! More devastating was when I would wake up to discover that the dream was for real.

Fortunately, a life of isolation has never felt safe to me, because I haven't been sick as long as some people, but those who have suffered from disease and disability for decades may find it difficult to want to leave the life that they know.

Illness may also be a haven for those accustomed to a life of self-sabotage, which also occurs because of past abuse. If, as children, we were berated and criticized and taught that we didn't deserve good things, in the absence of God or an influence to challenge those lies, we continue to lash ourselves with a life of defeat. We do this because it's what we know and are accustomed to. Believing that God wants a better life for us and that we are worthy of health, wealth and prosperous relationships, sits uncomfortably within our souls that, for a lifetime, have been fed other ideas. But God's words to us are not ours; they are far more optimistic and kind!

Believing God for a better life feels unsafe, so we cling to the safety of the life that we are used to and which sits in perfect alignment with our flawed perceptions of ourselves, because we think that we need to be safe, above all things. If we don't understand that we are worthy and that God is able to bring us into a life of true freedom, we may prefer to remain in our little cells of illness.

We must ask God to help us to get beyond our excuses and reveal to us whether sickness is a safe place for us to be, and if so, why. If it is, we must ask Him to dismantle the lies that keep us there and to embolden and empower us to get more involved in society. As uncomfortable as it may be at first, participating in a group activity or volunteering for a couple of hours a week at the local library can break us from the familiarity of disease and isolation (and supposing we are physically able to get out of the house). Challenging the lies that keep us imprisoned, as well as actively stepping out and doing what most frightens us, will free us.

God wants the best for us, which usually isn't the life that we have grown comfortable with. Just because it's what we know, doesn't mean that it's what He wants. He desires for us to be engaged with the world, to be involved in loving relationships with others, and to be healthy enough to actively participate in society.

→ *Disease Keeps Us from Taking Responsibility for Our Lives:* Some people cling to illness as a way to avoid taking responsibility for their lives. Past trauma prevents them from prevailing in relationships and in their life's work, so they avoid the hard work of change that is required of them to heal their trauma and which would enable them to prosper. They may believe that their wounds have marked them as permanent failures and so decide that their only alternative is to hide from situations that require them to face their ghosts.

Such people use disease as a cover-up for their inadequacies. They may say things like, "I can't remember my best friend's birthday because my disease has affected my memory." Or, "I lose my temper because this disease makes me do it!" Their complaints are valid, because disease truly does affect the memory and emotions, but the process is enabled by a lack of motivation to change, especially the thoughts.

Also, if physical healing brings us back into relationship with others, we may avoid it, if being in those relationships requires us to face our wounds and change aspects of ourselves that we don't have to deal with in our lives of isolation. Change is hard work, no matter how severe the trauma we have suffered. We are all sinful, flawed creatures, but unless we understand the power of the Holy Spirit to help us to overcome our trauma and change us, we may avoid that responsibility. If we don't believe we are able to change, then we will lack the motivation to do it.

Fortunately, God can do all things through us. It's not the depth of our wounding that matters, but rather our trust in His ability to change and empower us. If He created the earth, then He can enable us to face the responsibilities of life that frighten us and which we think we aren't able to fulfill. His power within us is infinite; it can change the hearts of all those around us and make it possible for us to do exceedingly, abundantly above and beyond all that we are capable of doing. If only we believe Him and step out in faith! We must make the decision to step out and do. He then takes our decision and our "do" and runs with it.

I recently attended a conference in which an international minister, Leif Hetland, spoke of how God has used Him to touch the hearts of nearly a million people around the world with Jesus' love. His life is a testimony to how brightly God's Spirit can shine in just one person. If only we know the strength of the power that resides within us and what He can accomplish through us! Many of us live defeated lives because we think that our success in life depends upon our own efforts. We may believe that God helps us, but we mostly expect to do life on our own. Yet, God can take the reins of our existence and accomplish through us infinitely more than what we are able to do on our own if we know that He is willing and able. Success in life isn't about trying as much as it is about trusting God; it isn't about striving, but instead, surrendering to His lordship. When we are able to do this, we find ourselves more empowered to take on life's responsibilities.

→ *We Are Afraid To Trust God for Good Things:* God showed us how much He loves us through Jesus' work on the Cross. If we can take hold of and meditate upon that marvelous event in history, and know that because He sent His only begotten Son to die for us, we can also believe Him to give us all that we need—which doesn't mean a life of destruction, depression and desolation. The devil comes to "steal and kill and destroy", but Jesus came "that they (we) may have life, and have it abundantly." (John 10:10) Especially in soul, mind and spirit.

We must take our hope one step beyond, and believe wholeheartedly that He will lift us out of our pits if we trust Him. In the meantime, we must declare His promises of health and life abundant, even if at first, they feel untrue to our hearts.

When symptoms threaten to rip to you shreds, speaking and meditating upon His promises may be the last thing you want to do. Because in your day that follows like every other, you are exhausted, in pain, and alone. You wonder why you should believe Him for anything different. Perhaps as a child, you believed Him for a better life, even when your alcoholic father beat your mother. Perhaps you believed Him when you never got asked to the school dance, thinking that surely someday, He would bring your prince to you and all would be okay. Perhaps you believed Him when you first got symptoms and thought, "He'll take care of this. I'll get better, I just know it." But when Daddy kept bruising Mommy, the prince found another princess, and a year of illness turned into three decades, you began to wonder whether God's promises were for you, after all.

Or perhaps as a child, every time you asked your parents for a doll or a train for Christmas, or permission to take up a new hobby or go to your neighbor Sally's slumber party, the answer was always "No." If your needs and desires were constantly denied, then you may have learned to believe that the good things in life were for other people. That you aren't deserving of them, since as a child, you seldom received your hearts' desires. So because you feel undeserving, it's difficult for you to believe that God wants to give you the gift of wellness or anything else that is good.

It may be too hard. It may hurt too much to hope. Your God has let you down, time and again. You fear that if you trust Him for healing, and He disappoints you, like a fragile vase, you just might shatter, once and for all. That prospect is terrifying. Perhaps you decide that it's better to hope, but to not take that hope too far into the realm of belief, because if what you hope for doesn't happen, you might renounce the God that you decided to give up the last shard of your soul to.

But is it better to live safe, but miserable, inside of your shell? You might as well risk trusting Him. He may not come through in the manner or time that you want Him to, but He promises—He promises!—to give a more abundant life to those that trust Him. He knows it's gut-wrenching. He knows what you've been through. But He wants you to close your eyes and take a flying leap off the cliff anyway, to see if you will believe Him to catch you.

What do you want to look at, anyway? Your ugly circumstances and the statistics of the unhealed around you, or God's promises? Which is more reliable? The evidence of what is seen, or He who has the power to heal you? Do you trust what you know, or who you know? Consider this: when you trust the "Who", the "What" of your life will change for the better!

The longer I follow God, the more I witness His miracles, and the more convinced I become that He wants to heal more people by His mighty hand. But He wants us to go beyond hope, and put our trust in Him, not our treatments or our circumstances.

Some of us don't understand the power of God to enable us to live victorious lives. We may try for a week or a month to trust Him, but when our circumstances or mindsets don't change, we quickly give up. Illness is an invitation for us to keep trying, because He may be the only hope that we have left. He wants to teach us to believe Him for a life of prosperity and victory, the process of which happens, paradoxically, when we are so desperate for a different life that we will do anything, including completely renouncing our wills to Him so that He can accomplish His work in us.

He is a kind, compassionate God who wants us to be well. He may use medicine as part of our healing process, but medicine doesn't cure all things. Only He can heal, lead, guide, and redefine us, from the inside out!

God is in the diamond business, and if we trust Him with all of our heart, He will clean the dirt from us and smooth our rough edges, so that we sparkle and shine as never before. We then receive the good things that life has denied us, and not because God never intended to give us the jewels of our hearts, but because He has made us into the jewels of His heart!

→ *We Feel Unworthy of God's Gift of Health:* God's promises of healing may mean little to those who believe themselves to be unworthy of His gifts. Feelings of unworthiness, or even worthlessness, can result from being taught early in life that we have no value, and from not knowing how much God loves us.

When I was really sick with Lyme, I used to envision Jesus, holding out a gift-wrapped package to me, with the words "health and life" stamped across them. While I could see the gift, I couldn't stretch out my arms to receive it. I knew it was there, but I couldn't touch it.

No, seriously, Jesus, I would think. This is for somebody else. Somebody who loves you more, who believes in You more, who doesn't have all of these intellectual roadblocks to healing. Besides, I've suffered far too much and for far too long. Health can't be your will for me.

That's honestly where I was, just a few years ago. Fortunately, God has slowly removed the lies that have kept me from believing that I don't deserve His gifts.

How do we receive God's gift of healing if we feel unworthy of it? Books and well-meaning Christians often say, "Well, if Christ died for us, then that makes us worthy." No doubt. He paid the price, so there is nothing we can do to make ourselves worthy, because He made us worthy by His work on the Cross and His great love for us. But this is just theology to those for whom God's love hasn't made it past the front door of their minds, and for those who mentally assent to Calvary but who can't quite figure out why God's sacrifice made them good enough.

"God loves you." People tell us. Oh, okay. We think. Well, that's great, isn't it? It would be nice if that knowledge would make it past the intellect though, into our hearts!

The belief that we aren't worthy of health (or other good things) sometimes masquerades as, and manifests in, other harmful beliefs, thought patterns, and actions, all of which function to sabotage our well-being and make us conclude that God's gift of healing isn't really for us.

For example, do you tell yourself that you're going to be sick forever, because your lifelong track record of health has been shoddy? The belief might be based on reason and solid circumstantial evidence, but careful—reason is sometimes a crafty disguise for self-sabotage and feelings of unworthiness, as I have learned.

Do you imagine a future of financial poverty and struggling to meet ends meet, because illness has vanquished your savings and you can't work? A logical concern...but did anyone in your past ever deny you basic material needs, or make you feel as though your needs didn't matter? Could it be that you are living out a destiny based on what somebody else thought you needed or deserved?

What about your relationships? Do others treat you poorly because of your disease? Do they challenge the notion that you are as sick as you say, or refuse you emotional or financial support when you really need it? Has this become your justification for becoming a recluse and avoiding relationships while in the throes of disease? Or did the isolation and loneliness precede your disease, and now your symptoms have become your soul's way of communicating that it's safer to live a solitary life?

Yes, illness is isolating. Perhaps you can't get out and about as much. You may have no money to spend on dinners with friends and family. Sadly, loved ones of the sick often live with their heads in the sand and their hearts out to lunch when it comes time for them to care for those that they are supposed to sacrificially love. The vow, "In sickness and in health" goes out the window when wives and husbands are left to fight their battles alone, as often happens when one partner becomes chronically ill.

On the other hand, it's pretty easy to use disease as an excuse to keep weak and wavering spouses, siblings and friends at bay. "Of course they don't care!" you might think. If they did, they would help you pay for your medications, rub your shoulders or take you to the doctor. So you hide, because, true to your lifelong story of rejection, these people, like those that made you or grew you into adulthood, aren't safe, or at least mature enough to give up their right to themselves in order to help you.

But why do you hide? Is it really because your loved ones aren't that loving? Maybe, but maybe you also needed for them to go away, because in the end, even the most perfect of imperfect love stings, and becomes too reminiscent of those who wounded or abused you in earlier years. Your subconscious may tell you that it's better to remain isolated by disease, even though consciously, you want to be healed, so that you can be in relationships again.

Don't be fooled. Our conscious mind often operates at odds with our subconscious mind. Both can be fabulous liars, by the way, and while the subconscious may want to protect the soul against getting hurt by allowing sickness to dominate the body, its methods are flawed. Hiding and making excuses for a half-assed life of survival have never freed anyone. Perhaps sickness has kept us from getting into further trouble by keeping us out of the world, but it hasn't healed us and it never will.

Then there are our conscious minds, which live in utter denial of the true reason for our disease. Okay, so some of us are sick strictly because of genetics or environmental factors; some pathogen, toxin, or accident stole our health from us. We may heal when given the appropriate remedy, but there are others for whom the remedies don't work, because harmful belief systems or traumas keep them mired in disease.

Often, the most pernicious and prevalent of these is that we don't believe that we deserve to be well, but we are often unaware that this belief exists, unless a wise friend, counselor, or God Himself, points it out to us.

If you have this belief, you may not recognize it for what it is. You may instead argue that you don't have money for treatments and that there is no cure for your disease. Or maybe you feel that nobody loves you, so you figure you might as well give up. These are all lies that Satan would have you believe. And as part of his song, he tells you that you might as well just lie down and die, because there's nothing you can do to change your lot in life.

On the other hand, perhaps you don't fight, because deep down, a voice is hissing, "You're not worth it!"Believing that God wants to give you life abundant seems laughable. Even if God desired that for you, you think that He wouldn't bestow it upon you in the form of a miracle.

Or maybe knowing that millions of people in the world die of AIDS, malnutrition, war, and all the rest, leads you to conclude that miracles are for a minority, if they happen at all.

Is this what you have learned to believe, because that's what you see around you? Because that's what you read in the news and what you witness in your family? Perhaps you think that disease and death are just the reality of life, and if God wanted to intervene in the lives of and heal those who get sick and die young, then He would have done it by now. But these are just comfortable beliefs for those who feel unworthy of health—indeed, of life.

Or maybe you believe that God heals—everybody in your church except you! Or that He heals nobody, because if He did, you would have seen somebody receive a miracle by now. Or that He extends healing only on occasion, to what you believe are His faith-filled pets and other random favorites. It may be easier to take medication and suffer a lifetime of pain, fatigue and bondage to depression, than dare believe that God wants to give you an amazing gift. Rain falls upon the murderer and the sanctified, selfless soul alike, and sometimes even more upon the selfless soul, right? Believing scares you. To risk another person—never mind the Creator of the universe, smashing your heart and your hope to smithereens again—feels akin to jumping off a cliff.

If you have such thoughts, you may want to ask yourself whether deep down, feelings of worthlessness or fears of rejection are governing your beliefs.

Perhaps the voice of rejection sings to you, "Don't believe God for healing because He might let you down! Don't believe Him for anything good, much less healing, because He isn't for real and even if He were, He wouldn't heal you, of all people!"

Worthlessness and unworthiness wear other faces, but their end result is the same; Jesus stands before you with a gift, but you can't take it, because you don't believe that it's meant for you.

How Do We Realize Our Worth Before God?

I don't know. The answer isn't the same for everyone. While I have seen God wipe away years of pain in an instant, this isn't how it usually works. In Chapter Seven, I discuss the methods that He sometimes uses to demonstrate how much He values and love us, and which He has used to heal me of my emotional trauma.

Take heart; there is a way out of every harmful belief that we've adopted, because God is bigger than our trauma and all that keeps us from His promises. He wants us to give us the gift of health even more than we want to receive it, and will guide us into all truth so that we can receive that gift. We must only take His hand, surrender and trust Him to show us the way.

We Fixate on Symptoms

Fixating on symptoms can become a way of life for the chronically ill. When burning nerve pain in your limbs, brain fog and fatigue scream for your undivided attention, they are difficult to ignore—

especially if you spend most of your time alone and have little else to distract you. Even focusing on God can be a challenge when symptoms are fierce. Yet, sadly, the adage that we are what we think is, to some degree, true. We become what we focus on, and if symptoms are the focus of our lives, depression and despair will follow. If they don't, then concentrating on the symptoms will ensure that they stay with us. One of the physicians that I interviewed for my second book, Dr. Steve Harris, who has treated thousands of Lyme disease patients, says that the people who experience the most healing from Lyme are those, "Who can focus on the disease (in order to adequately treat it) but not make it the focus of their lives."

Those severely disabled by chronic illness or an injury may have a more difficult time not making symptoms the focus of their lives. The more severe the symptoms, the harder they become to ignore. Also, in the absence of activities or people to spend time with, the sick often become stuck in a mindset of disease that becomes incredibly difficult to break. This hinders healing. It's important to strike a balance in our thinking, which is, unfortunately, harder to do than say.

So how do we focus upon God and His promises of healing if symptoms have been our food for thought for years? It's not easy, but with God's Spirit, all things are possible, and the more we choose to stay our eyes upon Him, the easier it will become to mind our thoughts.

It starts with baby steps, such as reading uplifting books that have nothing to do with disease, watching funny movies, or pursuing hobbies, such as painting or gardening, which distract the mind in a positive way. Playing beautiful, inspiring music feeds the soul, as does learning to meditate upon God and His promises and speaking those aloud. Resisting the temptation to complain or talk about our diseases with others is important, since complaining feeds our focus on symptoms and encourages self-pity. Sometimes we need a shoulder to cry on, but we need to be careful to not make discussions about disease the focus of our lives. Yes, illness is tragic, but magnifying the pain doesn't make it any less so. Besides, self-pity and complaining can be addictive and toxic.

The mouth is a powerful tool for shaping reality, and whatever we confess often becomes our reality. Earlier, I explained why it's important to speak God's Word, but in reality, all of our words matter. If we speak bitter words, they will feed our souls with anger. If we speak words of kindness, our hearts become lighter and softer. If we speak words of sickness, we will focus upon our symptoms and remain stuck in a mindset of disease. So, we must find other topics of conversation, even if our existence seems to be about little more than treatments and suffering through symptoms. We must ask God to help us to be more mentally tough, and to take every thought captive.

By itself, willpower is rarely sufficient to change a mind accustomed to meditating upon symptoms, but those of us who embrace the Holy Spirit have a power greater than ourselves living inside of us to help us. With practice and perseverance, we can change the negative and ugly into the positive and beautiful. But don't give up and beat yourself up when, some days, you slip up and complain for three hours about how poorly you feel. When you're sick, there's no greater challenge than speaking words of optimism. Yet, the effort is worth it, because over time, your thinking patterns may change if you are diligent and keep your eyes on the One who promises to deliver you. And as you focus your gaze upon Him instead of your symptoms, you will find yourself better able to believe Him for a healing miracle.

We Negate Our Faith by Our Words and Actions

If we agree that God wants us to be well, but negate that belief with words and actions of doubt, it reduces the strength of our convictions. For example, if we proclaim that it's His will to heal us, but focus constantly on our symptoms, or fret over whether a particular treatment is working, then our attention becomes fixated upon the very thing that we want to get rid of, rather than His promises. If, in our discouragement, we negate our faith with words like, "I wonder if I will ever be well?" or, "Is this all that God has for me?" it weakens our belief in His promises.

Of course, it's difficult to not utter words of doubt when symptoms are fierce, or when, despite our prayers, nothing seems to change. It doesn't help when our loved ones chastise us for our apparently delusional and desperate belief in the supernatural, and instead ask for details about our symptoms or a commentary about our current treatment regimen. Fortunately, God always forgives our moments of weakness and struggle, and can teach us a lot through them. He knows how hard it is. He doesn't expect us to be perfect, but because His Spirit is perfect, He will help us to cultivate a new mindset. It takes time.

Removing roadblocks of doubt requires strategizing our conversations and considering what we will say to others when they ask us how we are feeling. We shouldn't lie, but for every time that we confess that we feel bad, we should follow that with an affirmation of belief that God is healing us. If we are accustomed to negativity and speaking words of pessimism about our condition, we must come up with replacements for our complaints. It isn't an overnight thing, but resisting the urge to solicit sympathy from others or complain about how poorly we feel, even inwardly, can build our faith. For every discouraging thought we have, we should have an encouraging one at the ready to replace it. It's essential to make a list of the most common lies and complaints that we tell ourselves and others, and then come up with (and practice) positive statements to replace those. This is especially important if our suffering forms the basis of our relationships with others. If we have friends or family with caregiver tendencies, our relationship with them may be sustained by their need for us to have a problem, and by our need to complain about that problem. These alliances can be difficult to break, especially if they have been life long, because the continuance of the relationship has become dependent upon our suffering. Finding a new basis for the relationship requires brainstorming new topics of discussion, and refusing to give in to the need to whine about our latest and greatest symptom. If this doesn't work, we may need to distance ourselves from those who encourage our complaining, at least until we have become firmly rooted in new patterns of thought and speech.

For example, when people ask you how you are, if your habitual response is to say that you are tired, in pain, or just "hanging in there", you may want to instead say that you are well. You may not feel well, but responding with a negative comment about your physical or mental wellbeing will incite others to probe you for more information on your suffering. Before you know it, you are focusing upon your symptoms again! If your life has been consumed by disease, it may be difficult to find new topics of conversation. Reading books and magazines, watching television programs or You Tube videos on subjects that have nothing to do with disease can provide new food for talk. It takes practice, and you may want to brainstorm a list of new topics of conversation, so that you won't be tempted to fall into habitual patterns of unprofitable chatter.   Remember your passions and interests pre-illness, and consider ways to get involved in those again. If you used to travel, for instance, spend time reading about the places that you would still like to visit. Take an interest in the people and history of those places, by perusing blogs and articles on the Internet. If you used to be involved in a humanitarian cause, such as rehabilitating women from their lives of prostitution, you may find other ways to remain involved in that cause from home. Researching for an organization that helps women to recover their lives may be one way that you do this.   By getting involved in new activities, you then find that you have new things to talk about with others.

It's also good to ask God for an awareness of when you're meditating upon harmful beliefs, and speaking unhelpful words, because it's easy to let them slither through the mind and the mouth without you questioning whether they belong there.

I have found that I have good intentions of meditating upon and speaking words of truth, but unless I pray daily and ask God to point out when I start falling into a trap of pessimism, I forget to do this. Plus, at times, it's a huge effort and I get lazy or overwhelmed. But I'm also motivated by the fact that I can't afford the laziness; my happiness and health in this world depend upon it.

Cultivating an awareness of our thoughts and words, challenging the content of what gets put into our brains and replacing it with new content, is the first important step to removing our doubts about healing. During times of deep depression, challenging the thoughts may feel like a superhuman endeavor. We know that it's better to exchange our pessimism for positivity, but we may be so discouraged that we lack the motivation to do this. During such times, we must go to God and ask Him to fill our head with His thoughts, not ours, even if, at that moment, we don't think we will believe a word that He says; even if we are tempted to think, "Why speak God's promises of healing? It never works, it's all a lie, and God doesn't want me well..." Of course, such thinking is the result of the enemy of our souls planting some foul seed into our brains. But if we're depressed, these words may feel more real to us than any others that God or others would feed us. Yet, if we can manage to halt such thoughts in their tracks and grasp onto some better ones, it will benefit us. Little by little, as we practice challenging the harmful beliefs that get stuck in our brains, we gain an ever-increasing ability to refute them and replace them with truth. Biochemical dysfunction in the brain makes victory in this area more difficult, but it's worth pursuing, as over time, meditating upon truth also alters the biochemistry, just as healing the brain with medicine does. Again, our success doesn't depend upon us doing everything right; but rather, upon us taking God's hand and being willing to let Him pick us up after we fall, no matter how many times we hit the ground in defeat.

We Harbor Unforgiveness Against Ourselves, God and Others

For years, I was furious with God without realizing it. My anger mostly manifested as a lack of desire to pray or spend time with Him, a vague uneasiness when I did, or as words of resentment whenever life didn't go my way.

As a child, I often prayed, but it seemed God seldom responded to my petitions. Because of this, I began to build a wall around my heart. I still have an old diary from my childhood. One of the lines in it reads,

"God made me ugly, stupid and unpopular!" I came to this conclusion because I was a shy, slow, awkward child who didn't have many friends and who had little notion of how to do school and life with other kids. People made fun of my clothes and huge blue eyes and God did nothing (apparently) to change my misperceptions about myself. Of course, at the time I had only a vague awareness of what God's love looked like in practical terms, and even less of an idea about how He redeems a broken life, so my expectations were flawed. In any case, I decided that if God wasn't going to answer my prayers, then I wasn't going to talk to Him anymore. I was a young teenager when I made that decision, and I stuck by it until age twenty-eight. Sure, I thought about God in the interim, and made half-hearted prayer requests on occasion, but my image of Him had been distorted, and I mostly believed that He didn't care about me. How sad that I missed out on experiencing His love for so many years!

The image that I had developed of God as a child continued into my adulthood, and even after I consented to handing my life over to Him, more years passed before I was able to see Him in a different light. As this light shone into my heart, I discovered how my unforgiveness towards Him had become a barrier to understanding His love.

If we can't forgive God, we may believe that He needs to punish us with disease, especially if our image of Him is that of a drill sergeant who is keen on whipping His Creation into shape. If we believe that punishment is what He wants to give us, and that this is what we deserve, then His love can't flow through us and our cells will cling to disease.

When we forgive God for not meeting our expectations, we have a greater capacity to fellowship with Him and believe Him for good things, including health. It's okay to tell God when we feel let down by Him, and confess that we don't like what He's doing in our lives, as long as we also ask Him for a heart to receive the truth about His purposes and love for us.

He can't heal us if we harbor bitterness against Him, and when we refuse to forgive Him, our bodies hold on to that unforgiveness in the form of symptoms. Resentment and rage don't just live in the brain, but in every cell, tissue and organ of our bodies.

Practitioners of Chinese medicine believe that the organs harbor specific emotions. For instance, rage is often stored in the liver, and fear is held in the kidneys. Both of these emotions can result from unforgiveness. Because God has given us free will, He can't spontaneously remove that unforgiveness. We must choose to let it go, and when we do, the accompanying emotions get released from our cells.

Acknowledging anger against God may be difficult, because religion has taught us that we aren't supposed to be angry at Him. Instead, we mask our disappointment in Him with flowery prayers, while stuffing our true emotions. The Bible admonishes us to thank God and praise Him, but we must also be honest with Him, because He wants a real relationship with us. He wants us to share the contents of our heart with Him, even if those contents contain sharp edges and cutting words. He can handle our pain and isn't going to send us to the depths of Hell for our anger. He knows we're human, but He doesn't appreciate hypocrisy any more than we do, and we behave as hypocrites when we praise Him with words, but secretly harbor bitterness against Him. Yet His love is larger than our trauma and He will help us to forgive Him, if we are willing.

Similarly, we must examine our hearts to discern whether we have any unforgiveness towards ourselves. We may be flagellating ourselves for things that we have done or failed to do over the decades of our lives, and memories of those things are bruising our battered bodies. We may be chastising them for betraying us and for not being able to function normally. Or we may be mentally whipping ourselves for hurting our children and scaring our spouses away with our cutting words. We may be living with regrets over failed dreams, and despising ourselves for not having made better choices in life. We may be blaming ourselves for our illnesses and rolling in remorse for not having done anything to prevent them.

It isn't holy to beat ourselves up over our mistakes. It isn't humble to make disparaging comments about ourselves or constantly regret the past. God doesn't approve of us rehashing what we should, or could, have done. Neither does He smile when we rip His Creation (ourselves) apart with our words. We are "fearfully and wonderfully made" (Psalm 139:14), and it's time that we started appreciating and accepting who God has made us to be. Some people think that God focuses mostly upon our flaws, but God is ever-gazing at us with eyes of wonder and joy. He is proud of His Creation and of the workmanship of His hands. We are His treasures, made in His perfect image. We are the "apple of His eye." (Psalm 17:8)!

God wants us to recognize our sins and repent of them, but once we have done that, He wants us to kick them out of our memory. He has canceled our debts, and not forgiving ourselves is the same thing as saying that Jesus' sacrifice on the Cross wasn't sufficient to atone for all of our mistakes. It's like saying that what we have done is above and beyond any atoning sacrifice that God could ever make for us and we therefore don't deserve to be forgiven. There is no humility in saying, "What I did was so awful, I just can't forgive myself, even though I know that God forgives me." Because when we refuse to forgive ourselves, we disregard Jesus' work and declare our standard to be higher than God's. But who are we to set the standard? If God has forgiven us, we need to forgive ourselves. Not just for our sake, but for His and for the sake of those who love us. Self-flagellation never benefits anyone.

Finally, we must forgive others for the ways in which they have hurt us. Many of the chronically ill have been deeply betrayed by friends and family. People who were supposed to love us abandoned us when we became sick, or sometime along the way, got fed up with our suffering and couldn't handle it anymore. They may have turned a blind eye to our financial needs, ignored us in our isolation, refused to comfort us when we needed it, or denied us when we asked for a helping hand around the house. It can be difficult to forgive those who weren't there for us when we most needed them. Few things cause greater pain to the soul than when we bleed, are desperate for help, and the whole world seems to walk away. It destroys our faith in humanity and confuses us, especially when those loved ones have, in sunnier seasons, always been there for us.

Over the past five years, I have seen longstanding marriages end after one of the partners contracted Lyme disease. I have witnessed friends losing friends, parents ignoring their children, and children ignoring their parents in their distress. I have been ignored and rejected myself. It's funny how the people that we most love and whom we most thought would be there for us in our suffering, are sometimes those that vanish from the scene when the going gets rough. I have also found that those whom we don't expect to be there for us, lesser friends and acquaintances, are sometimes more supportive than spouses, close friends and other family members.

We must give grace to those who fail us. They are human, and like all humans, have a limited capacity for suffering. It isn't that they don't want to love us; they may not be able to. Their love resources are finite, and the less love that they have received from God themselves, the less they have to give us. And who knows if they aren't carrying around a tremendous burden of guilt for what they weren't able to do or be for us?

It can take months, even years, to forgive our loved ones for betraying us. We must ask God, day after day, to heal us as we affirm to Him our desire to forgive those who have wronged us. We may not experience any change in our feelings for a long time, but if we persevere, He who is faithful promises to restore us, because only He can release us from our prisons of rage. We make the decision to forgive, but He then honors our decision and heals our emotions. Over time, and as we continually affirm our desire to forgive, our hearts become mended.

Also, it has been said that when we forgive, we release a prisoner and that prisoner is us. We hold nobody captive by our hatred except ourselves, and as the popular TV evangelist Joyce Meyer once said, "Not forgiving another is like taking poison and hoping that the other person will die."

Besides, the Bible commands us to forgive others as God has forgiven us. If Jesus gave up His life as a propitiation for our sins; if He was beaten and bled to death so that we might be reconciled to God and live in eternity with Him, then we owe it to Him to release others from the injustices that they have committed against us.

May He give us all the ability to forgive our loved ones, just as Jesus forgave His friends, even though they all left Him (the most perfect and loving of all human beings) to die alone on a Cross! May the amazing love that Jesus showed His friends and even those who murdered Him penetrate our hearts and spirits, too.

We Live in Ingratitude towards God

Sometimes, ingratitude blocks our healing. If we aren't thankful for what God has already given us, then why should He give us anything else? If we fail to recognize the gifts that He has generously bestowed upon us, everything from the food on our plates to the roof over our heads and the gift of salvation that we have in Christ Jesus, then why should He heal us, if we won't be thankful for that gift? Like people, God appreciates it when we acknowledge His gestures of kindness towards us with a thankful heart.

In my travels to over fifty nations, I have observed that people in wealthier nations tend to have a greater spirit of entitlement towards God. They expect things from Him, and become bitter when they don't get what they want. Perhaps it's because people in first-world countries are accustomed to comfort and an abundance of material possessions, more so than those who have to scrape and save for toilet paper or a son's birthday cake.

When I lived in Costa Rica, I participated in a weekly Bible study that was held in an impoverished, somewhat dangerous neighborhood of San Jose. The people who attended the study lived in moldy homes with cheap, torn and broken furniture. Their clothes were well-worn and many subsisted on little more than rice, beans and cheap soda pop.

Few people had cars, and those that did were constantly repairing theirs. My friends that lived there seldom had money for recreational activities, although occasionally, they might attend a dollar movie. Yet, their attitude towards God was always one of thankfulness. They praised Him continually for His provision. My good friend Roxana, whose car was always breaking down, and who routinely had the electric company threatening to turn her lights off because she couldn't pay her bill, often proclaimed that God always met her every need. I would think, "Seriously? Doesn't God know that you need lights in your house? Doesn't God know that you need a car for your catering business?" Her perspective challenged my notion of what it means to be provided for by God, but her attitude of gratitude, along with that of other people in the neighborhood, showed me that riches don't make a person thankful. In fact, they may do the opposite, and create a spirit of entitlement in those to whom they are given.

I encourage you to take two minutes every morning to thank God for His gifts to you. Even if you don't feel thankful, speaking words of gratitude can remove the temptation to entertain a spirit of entitlement, which leads to bitterness towards God. Sometimes, our feelings change for the better when we simply decide to thank God, even if at first we don't feel like it. It's even better if we can thank Him through the storms of life, because when we do, their power to overwhelm us gets broken. It also keeps us out of the clenches of self-pity.

We Have a Closed Mind about God

Some people don't receive from God because they refuse to open their eyes, listen with their ears, and receive His truths with a willing heart. According to the Bible, God has revealed Himself to every human being, but not everyone has acknowledged Him. Romans 1:18-20 states: "For the wrath of God is revealed from heaven against all ungodliness and wickedness in those who, by their wickedness, suppress the truth. For what can be known about God is plain to them, because God has shown it to them. Ever since the creation of the world, his eternal power and divine nature, invisible though they are, have been understood and seen through the things he has made. So they are without excuse; for though they knew God, they did not honor him as God or give thanks to him, but they became futile in their thinking, and their senseless minds were darkened. Claiming to wise, they became fools; and they exchanged the glory of the immortal God for images resembling a mortal human being or birds or four-footed animals or reptiles."

Ultimately, either we choose relationship with Him or we do life without Him. No matter our history of trauma or mental dysfunction, He has said that He has made Himself known to all of us through the things that He has made. So in the end, our ability to receive from Him boils down to a decision to acknowledge Him, as well as our willingness to be open to the ways in which He works in the world.

Once we acknowledge Him, we must realize that He seldom runs the universe as we expect, and His ways don't conform to the dimensions of our proverbial God boxes. They may seem bizarre, implausible, or even frightening, and when it comes to healing, out of a need to find safety with the familiar, we may shun the idea that He performs miracles, signs and wonders today. As Bill Johnson, pastor of Bethel church in Redding, CA, writes in his book, *When Heaven Invades Earth,* "While few would admit it, the attitude of the Church in recent days has been, 'If I'm uncomfortable with something, it must not be from God.'" Here, he is referring to the ways in which the Holy Spirit manifests in people, and how people reject Him when He shows up in ways that they are unaccustomed to. While Bill isn't specifically referring to healing here, this concept may also be applied to supernatural healing.

God can't heal us if we won't receive Him on His terms. Religion and life may have given us flawed expectations about how He operates in the universe, but we must be willing to revise what religion, experience or our mothers have taught us.

Those who have a closed mindset can witness miracles, read about Jesus' miracles, and still not believe that God heals today. In Matthew

13, Jesus describes people whose hearts and minds are closed to truth. In verse 15, He says, "For this people's heart has grown dull, and their ears are hard of hearing, and they have shut their eyes; so that they might not look with their eyes, and listen with their ears, and understand with their heart and turn—and I would heal them."

Maybe bitterness over the death of a loved one has kept you from believing that He won't save your next family member from the grave. Maybe you don't believe, because just as many Christians die from disease as non-Christians. (And while this may be true, how many Christians in developed countries believe in the commonality of miracles? Would it change the statistics if they did?)

I encourage you to release your fears and let God out of your proverbial box. He manifests His power and love in creative, amazing ways, but these ways are sometimes strange to us. We shouldn't limit Him just because we fear the supernatural and/or our church has taught us not to pursue signs and wonders. You may have had a relative that believed for a miracle from God and died, but just because God didn't do things according to how that person thought He would, doesn't mean that He doesn't yet heal multitudes. Just because the Church has taught you that Jesus doesn't heal today, doesn't mean that this is accurate theology. Just because the manifestations of the Spirit seem bizarre to you, doesn't mean that they aren't holy and true. God has some interesting ways of revealing Himself to people!

Chapter 6

Where Supernatural Healing Abounds

Miracles in Third-World Nations

I have lived in three countries besides the United States: Argentina, Costa Rica and the United Kingdom, and have spent extensive periods of time in others. I have also traveled to over fifty countries in Asia, Africa, Latin America, and Europe. My interest and knowledge of other cultures is relatively broad, and I've seen and heard of God doing great miracles in these places—including raising people from the dead!

A documentary video entitled "The Finger of God," reveals the ministry of a woman named Heidi Baker, who was called to the poorest country in the world, Mozambique, in 1995, to share God's love with others. Over the years, God has used her and people in her ministry to establish over 5,000 churches across the African continent and perform thousands of healing miracles.

Miracles are a primary way that Jesus, God the Father and the Holy Spirit introduce themselves to people in nations that have never heard about the God of Christianity. They do this so that the people in these places will know that there exists a powerful, kind and compassionate God in the universe who is real and cares for them. Manifestations of God's love through the supernatural, when combined with Jesus Christ's message, prove that He isn't just western white man's religious doctrine, but a God who loves and reveals Himself to all, in powerful ways.

In addition to healing miracles, God has also used Heidi Baker and people in her ministry to raise over 300 people from the dead! Included in the "Finger of God" documentary is the testimony of a man who was murdered, then raised from the dead by God's hand. After he was resurrected, he forgave his perpetrator. What a powerful demonstration of God's love and power on earth!

Other stories of healing and great miracles abound in underdeveloped countries, and while on mission trips to Guatemala, Colombia and Ecuador, I have spoken with people who have testified to God's power to supernaturally heal them when no medicine was available.

Supernatural healing happens more often in underdeveloped countries than in reason-based, first-world nations. This may be because in the latter, medicine is more accessible, confusion over God's will for physical healing abounds, and people are more complacent towards their Creator. I have observed that the impoverished in underdeveloped countries usually have greater faith in God and His ability to heal and provide—perhaps because they have no other choice. They must rely upon Him constantly, because they don't have jobs that pay the bills and neither do they have access to adequate medical care. They don't have 401K's, savings, and exposure to dozens of different theologies that distract, confuse and contradict the Bible. They read the Bible and they take God at His word, instead of over-analyzing the Scriptures and the doctrine of healing. They haven't been exposed to books that argue that God doesn't heal and which only serve to confuse North Americans and Western Europeans; neither have they been introduced to information that refutes God's provision for them. Innocence, simplicity, desperation for God, tragedy and financial hardship are catalysts for their faith and for receiving healing from God.

I have observed that faith in God's ability to work supernaturally seems to be weaker in societies of comfort, where reason, the intellect and senses are exalted above the supernatural and God's promises in the Bible. In such societies, people don't really know how much they need God because the majority of them still have food, shelter and access to medicine that, while far from perfect, still offers some hope for wellness. That hope feels more secure than depending upon a seemingly capricious God; an unknown entity, who only heals every once in awhile.

What if those of us who live in the most developed nations of the world began to believe Him for healing? What if our hope in medicine and our ability to heal ourselves got snatched out from under us? What if we truly had to rely upon Him minute-by-minute for our food and all that we need? Yes, the chronically ill may be more adept at relying upon God than those with greater health and resources because illness creates financial poverty. But because medicine yet extends a hand of hope to us, we hold out for a miracle in medicine instead of in God. Or if we don't, a lifetime of being conditioned to believe that God can't— or won't—heal us, keeps us from stretching out our hands to receive that healing. Those of us who have faith for healing sometimes negate that faith by praying the faith-destroying words, "If it be Thy will." By proclaiming such words, we introduce the possibility that God may not want us to be well. And if we haven't been healed yet, then in the dark recesses of our minds, we may assume that it's not God's will for us to be well, even though we strive to believe. While it's good to acknowledge and accept God's will in our lives, we should always claim His desire for our wholeness.

At a recent conference, evangelist Randy Clark, who has been used to share the love of God and heal thousands worldwide, seconded my belief that more miracles happen overseas than in the United States and other developed countries. At his meetings overseas, (on average) at least 80% of those who attend receive a healing! My understanding is that he believes this happens (at least in part) because people in wealthier nations have been indoctrinated to believe that God doesn't heal supernaturally, so it's more difficult for us to receive from Him.

Heidi Baker and her husband, Rolland, have written several books on their experiences in Africa. In one, *Expecting Miracles,* Heidi writes of her ministry, "How has Africa increased my faith? Where do I start? I see healing as I have never experienced in my life. This is where the gospel in Africa is ten times better than in the West! They are super desperate for the Word of God. They believe and they get healed."

So, according to Heidi, desperation for God and His Kingdom are also catalysts for receiving. People in African nations have few material comforts, and are often so broken by hardship that they readily receive from God. Wealth and resources have made people in developed countries complacent in their passion for God, and have fooled them into thinking that God's material gifts are what they most need, rather than His presence. Her book confirmed my suspicion that because most Africans can't rely upon the things of this world for their joy (some literally have nothing!) they readily rely upon God to meet all of their needs. As His presence fills them, they are healed because they truly know that He is the only One that can take away their pain.

As I mentioned earlier, my friend Troy, who has trod alongside me through the trenches of Lyme disease, was recently used by God to heal many people in Colombia. He has suffered from chronic Lyme disease for many years, yet God has been using him in Colombia to supernaturally heal others on a daily basis. As part of a recent email to me, he wrote:

"...Anyway, the miracles (here) are too many to list right now, but I am writing them down daily. This is blowing me away! God is so much bigger than we perceive Him to be. In the Bible, the children of Israel limited the Lord with their negative attitude towards healing. The Scriptures teach us to never do that, but instead, to declare the miracles that we have seen. Remember, they aren't mine or yours; they belong to our great God. Declare the (healing) testimonies (to others), because it's amazing how God will honor them. They are our delight and our counselors. Here, I am seeing people with arthritis being healed instantly, as well as those who suffer from problems in their colons, backs, kidneys, hearts, and other organs. As God uses me to heal others, it's as if I am doing nothing but declaring the testimonies and calling down His Kingdom (from Heaven). It's so easy because it's His strength and power doing the work, not mine."

Maybe if those of us in rich, reason-based nations witnessed more divine miracles, we would experience more of them in our lives. Maybe if every hospital, clinic and doctor in the United States vanished (not that we want them to!), we would open our hearts and minds to other avenues of healing. Maybe it's all about giving in to God, and allowing Him to color outside of our preconceived lines of truth. Maybe it's about desiring Him, above all things!

Chapter 7

How to Experience the Love of God

The real miracle that we receive from God is His love. When we have that, we have all things. Sometimes, God heals our bodies to show us how much He loves us, but at other times, we must believe in His love first in order to receive the healing in our bodies. It's difficult to believe God for a miracle if we don't believe that He loves us, because faith in His healing is based upon our faith in His love for us.

We Must See Him as a Person, Not a Religion

The Church has often made God into a set of rules to be followed instead of into a being to be loved. This is religion, not relationship with our Creator, and God intended the latter for us! Sadly, in the secular world, Christians are known more for what they are against instead of what they are for. Some point fingers at those with alternative lifestyles as they make a hullabaloo over homosexuality, pornography, drug addiction and abortion, thereby giving those who are involved in these things the idea that God rejects them. The Church often misses what I believe is our true sin—independence from God's life inside of us—and in its negligence has driven away droves of souls starving for His presence. Some churches exalt morality above loving communion with our Creator, but is morality what a relationship with God is supposed to be about? Following a prescribed set of rules in order to avoid Hell? Taking the recipe of salvation, which involves a) confessing that you are a sinner, b) repenting for being a sinner, and c) accepting Christ's gift of salvation? Put the recipe in the oven, and poof! You are saved? Yes, it's all that God requires of us to spend eternity with Him, and the elements are vital for a relationship with Him, but because they are sometimes presented as a formula, His love gets lost in the translation.

God sent Jesus to earth to show us what He is like, and most people who believe in Him get that part. God can be a good guy, as evidenced by Jesus' words, miracles and gentle touch upon humanity during the time that He walked the earth. But the biggest reason why Jesus came to earth was to pay for our evil deeds with His blood and suffering and make a way for us to come back into fellowship with God. That is, God the Father sent Jesus to earth as a ransom for our sins; to pay the price for our rebellion against Him, so that we might be reconciled to Him and live happily ever after with Him, as we experience His Heaven on earth!

It's like this: we screw up, and God the Father bears the burden for our mistakes and sends His only begotten Son to die for us. We do nothing but believe in Him and His sacrifice, and repent for doing life without Him. That is His amazing gift to us.

Jesus had to become a sacrifice for humanity because flawed, sinful human beings can't co-exist in relationship with a holy God unless their sins are atoned for. It's just a rule of the Heavenlies. Fortunately, Jesus' sacrifice makes us worthy of that relationship and of spending eternity with God. His sacrifice is also a powerful demonstration of how much He loves us.

Humanity has been in rebellion against God since the beginning of time by choosing to do life its own way and has made an abundant mess of the earth and all of its creatures in the process. So God, knowing that this would happen, had a plan since the creation of the universe. It's as if He said: "I know that My people are going to hurt, hate, and destroy one another and their environment. They will even hurt and hate me, the One who gave them life. But because I want them to have free will to do as they please, I will allow it. And I will send my beloved Son down to earth as a human, and sacrifice Him to make amends for their wrongs, because I love them dearly and I want them to be reconciled to Me. They will nail Him to a cross, but I will allow it, for their good and My glory. They will ridicule and spit on Him; beat, bruise and bleed Him to death, and I will turn my eyes away in grief, as my Son takes all of their sin upon Himself on that Cross. Every last ugly word they have uttered and will ever utter; every action that they have taken and will ever take to intentionally hurt, maim and kill others; every lust, greed and perversion, He will bear…

…And so I will forget that they ever hurt Me and the people that I created them to be in communion with. If only they choose to recognize what I am doing for them by allowing My Son to be crucified on a Cross! I will forget it all and take them to be with Me forever in a place of eternal love, beauty and joy. It will grieve me deeply to know that my Son will suffer so, but it will be worth it, because I desperately love My people. I will only ask that they repent for living their lives independently of me, and recognize that they have harmed themselves and others by doing so. Then I will ask them to acknowledge that I am paying the price for their mistakes. Their forgiveness will cost me my Son's life on earth, but I will suffer that hurt a thousand times over if it means that they will eventually come back to Me. Oh, may they surrender to Me, so that I may give them new life! Because this is the other part of the gift; I will send my Son to not only be a sacrifice for them, but also to give them a better life on earth by My Spirit, who will dwell in all who believe in Me. After Jesus is resurrected to Heaven, I will send the Spirit to My people, that they might have My life and all of the holiness, power and love that that entails, living inside of them."

This is Christianity: recognizing that we have sinned against our

Creator by not acknowledging Him and by choosing to do life our way instead of His. Then, accepting His sacrifice and surrendering to His mighty Spirit that dwells inside all who are willing to give their lives back to Him.

Christianity isn't about being good, following rules, or living a constrained life where God doesn't meet our needs. It's not about being judged for not meeting God's standards. It would be silly to think that we can meet the standards of a Holy God, anyway! A changed life of obedience results from surrendering to the Spirit, and is the byproduct of knowing God's love and responding to His Spirit within; it isn't the result of anxious striving or obligatory obedience. It's simply about a relationship of dependence upon the One who made us.

Romans 8:1 states, "There is therefore now no condemnation for those who are in Christ Jesus. For the law of the Spirit of life in Christ Jesus has set you (us) free from the law of sin and death." That is, God condemns nobody who has received Jesus as their Lord and Savior, and His Spirit has set us free from our old, sinful natures that are in bondage to the devil and a life of deception, defeat and destruction. Anyone who has received the Holy Spirit is no longer controlled by this old nature (although they may still choose to live by it). Instead, the Spirit empowers and guides us into a better life, one that ultimately brings wisdom, victory and joy, and according to His better ways, not ours.

If God desires to give us "life abundant" (John 10:10) by the Holy Spirit, then why do we resist Jesus Christ and His desire for us? Why do we resist the path of holiness, if it's ultimately supposed to bring us peace and knowledge of a love that's greater than anything we can ever experience on earth? Why, if it brings us into relationship with the only One who can give us the desires of our hearts?

Could it be because our minds have been darkened by the evil one? How about by religious hypocrites and false doctrine that has been preached and pounded into our brains by people who needed control or who valued being right over being loving? Or perhaps our understanding has been clouded by those who were supposed to love us early in life, but who instead abused us, so that now God's love seems synonymous with these false expressions of love (or lack thereof) that we have received in our lives. Maybe we have been turned away from truth because of the tragedies that we witness all around us; bodies broken by famine, disease and war. Or perhaps it's because of our culture, which popularizes relativism in religion and new age doctrine, both of which keep us from pursuing the path of Jesus. (But just because it's fashionable nowadays to believe that all paths lead to God, doesn't mean that there isn't one absolute truth about God that He wants us to discover. Not all Christians have this truth, either. They may attend church and read the Bible, but it doesn't necessarily mean that they know an iota about God or have a personal experience of Him. God speaks to people of all religions but this doesn't mean that all religions point to God. He lives in the hearts of those who are open to Him and His call upon their lives, but unless the message of the Cross reaches them in truth, and touches them in their innermost being, they may want nothing to do with Him.

Yet, if this God was willing to sacrifice His only begotten Son Jesus for our sake, then why believe in another God? I know of no other religion that has a God that is as loving, kind, merciful, faithful and marvelous as the God of Christianity, because no God has died for Creation as this One has, and no God offers us unconditional love, acceptance and eternal life, regardless of our behavior. Only this One does.

Do you believe that God would have sent His Son to die for you, if you had been the only human on earth? Those of us who believe in and understand the message of the Cross may yet believe Jesus' sacrifice to be a blanket gift for all of humanity. We may find it difficult to believe that He would stand before us with tears in His eyes, His blood pouring out, saying, "Here, look, I'm willing to die for you, and only you, see?" Why is that? Do we really think that little of ourselves, or of Him?

If the reality of the Cross doesn't touch us as a profound revelation of God's love for us, then it may take time for Him to erase from our hearts the false beliefs that we have about Him and ourselves, which have been chiseled there over a lifetime of tragedies.

Can the God of the universe overcome our harmful programming? Of course! If He gave up His life for us, wouldn't He also help us to be well in body, mind, and spirit? Why not keep praying for revelation as we study and meditate upon the marvelous work that He has accomplished for our sakes? Or at least talk to Him and see what happens? Maybe that's the greatest step of faith there is: to reach out to what we cannot see and discover that maybe, just maybe, there is someone there waiting for us.

I have noticed that whenever I pray and am able to meditate deeply upon the meaning of God's sacrifice, it helps me to see God as a person, not a religion, and realize my worth before Him. Especially when I consider the fact that had I been the only person on earth, He would have still died for me, and me alone! In such moments, it seems absurd to me that He would want anything for His children but a life of health and prosperity in Him.

Making the Jesus of the Bible the Jesus of Our Lives

I once asked a friend if he thought that God would heal everyone who asked for it. He said, "Well, if Jesus were here in the flesh today, do you think He would heal you?"

This question intrigued me. In my suffering, I have often considered how wonderful it would have been to have lived during Jesus' time, and known that if I had just touched the hem of His garment, that I would have been healed instantly. That all I would have had to do was follow Him and ask Him to heal me. He wouldn't have said No, I am sure, because He never denied anyone who came to him seeking wellness. He always showed great compassion towards all those whom He came into contact with. So if the same Spirit that worked miracles through Jesus still lives in His followers today, then why wouldn't He heal me today, either by His Spirit within me or through another anointed soul?

When my friend asked me this question, I realized that my personal Jesus wasn't the same Jesus of the Bible. My Jesus wasn't a Jesus of power, mercy or compassion. He was silent through my suffering; He watched me from afar, sympathetic to my plight but unwilling to do anything but provide me with some spotty guidance about which remedies to take. Sometimes, He was a Jesus that dangled a set of keys in front of me, as He waited for me to figure out which one would open the door to my prison. If I just tried harder, to do this or that, then He could set me free with a miracle.

My friend's question made me realize that I needed to re-vamp the way in which I viewed my Jesus. I had to learn that just because we can't see Him, doesn't mean that He doesn't dwell among us today and perform the same miracles as yesterday. The same Jesus who, over 2000 years ago, made food multiply and forgave sins; who comforted, taught and healed others, still wants to be involved in our lives. He wants to be our friend, counselor, comforter, encourager, provider, and healer; our everything! Most of all, He wants to know us and for us to know Him.

Undoubtedly, God allows hardship into the lives of His children, but is being sick God's definition of "life abundant?" Did the Jesus of the Bible ever deny comfort or healing to those who sought Him for it? Not once did He say to those who crossed His path, "Suffer this sickness, because it's good for you." Or, "You are worthless and deserve to be sick." Or... (fill in the blank with your own mental script!) Sadly, the enemy of our souls often convinces us that the evil visited upon our lives is necessary for us to be able to grow in love.

If the Jesus of the Bible is kind, wise, loving and the healer of all man's ills, and if Jesus represents the most complete revelation of God on earth, today, yesterday and forever, then why shouldn't this God be the One that we have a relationship with today? Instead of the God who is nothing but a skewed reflection in our minds of the punishing and flawed authority figures of our past?

Hearing the Voice of God in Prayer

Searing pain in my hips and back sometimes awakens me at four a.m. My body vibrates as Lyme bugs pluck my nerves like a frazzled guitar, and I stumble out of bed to take a shot of magnesium, swallow a handful of almonds to curb my crashing blood sugar, and rub some Biofreeze ointment on my back so that I can return to my nightmares and fitful slumber for another four hours.

In the meantime, the broken record in my brain begins its usual litany of curses. "Life sucks, doesn't it? Why, just look at you! Thirty-something years old and you can't even sleep through the night without having to put all that junk into your body. Your bones creak like an old woman's. If it's this bad now, imagine what you're going to feel like in twenty years! Imagine the mess that those Lyme spirochetes will have made of you by then. Your insides will have all kinds of holes. Your tissues and organs will look like shredded garments."

If I'm really feeling bad and allow my mind to be lazy (which it often is at 4 a.m.), then my unguarded thoughts descend further into a pit of pessimism. "God is a liar. He has never given you the desires of your heart. For years, you have believed Him to heal you, and look! You are as sick as ever. He loves you but He can't heal you because you don't have enough faith. Besides, He needs to teach you a lesson through your disease. He needs you to understand how much He loves you, but since you don't seem to get that, you'll be stuck in this pit of Hell forever. Forget ever getting married or having a purpose beyond writing some book on Lyme disease every few years. Your lot in life is to be sick, isolated and impoverished...forever! You think God loves you? Well, it's a strange kind of love, isn't it? What kind of God would curse His children with disease?"

And all that within the first two minutes that I am awake, finding my way to the porcelain bowl and scrambling to the kitchen to swallow ten thousand pills so that I can forget my pain and go back to sleep!

When symptoms are fierce and I'm half-asleep, reigning in these insidious thoughts is difficult. Those who have never experienced neurological illness cannot fathom the extraordinary challenge that it is to "take every thought captive to obey Christ" (2 Cor. 10:5), no matter that the Holy Spirit helps us in our weaknesses. Many of us don't realize the magnitude of the power of the Spirit within us to overcome and even those of us that do may have a stronger battle against the flesh and the enemy than those with healthier minds and bodies. I know because I witness a huge difference in my ability to "take every thought captive" during periods of greater health, when treatments aren't knocking me to the ground.

Yet God's Spirit can overcome all things, including our broken bio-chemistry, although our failed attempts to overcome our negative thinking may cause us to conclude that this isn't so. It may seem that no matter how many happy words we utter, our mountains of depression and anxiety refuse to move. We try, we cry, we pray, we read the Bible, we recite healing verses and yet...the trauma wins. Or so it seems.

Eight years ago, when I surrendered my life to God, I told Him that I would do anything for Him, if He just gave me peace. At that time, my anxiety and depression were off the charts. I suffered from obsessive thoughts. I feared anything and everything. I had panic attacks and developed agoraphobia (anxiety of being in certain places). I couldn't drive on the highway, get on an airplane, or watch catastrophic news on TV. Fear of dying of a heart attack gripped me at every turn, and tears were my daily food. This hell lasted for several years.

I prayed and experienced moderate peace, but only for as long as I remained in prayer. Three years later, I discovered I had Lyme disease, and as God used medicine, nutrition, counseling and vitamin supplements to heal my brain and body, the anxiety began to diminish. In the meantime, my doctor put me on a strong anti-depressant, which, within three days, miraculously removed the fiercest of the anxiety symptoms that I had suffered from for several years.

I was discouraged. If the Holy Spirit within me was supposed to overcome all things, then why was a drug doing more for my peace than the Spirit?

"There's something missing in your faith walk," one well-meaning friend said to me during this agonizing period of my life. "You should have more joy than this."

His words cut me. I felt judged and I wished he understood what was happening to me. But at the time, I didn't even know what was going on. I hadn't yet discovered that I had Lyme disease.

In hindsight, I realized that God had been at work, even though His touch upon my life hadn't felt like much at the time. I expected a healing miracle when I gave my life to Him, because I had seen people freed from their anxiety and grief in an instant once they decided to follow Him. But for some good reason, He allowed me to walk a different, more difficult, path.

So, instead of an instant miracle, He directed me to do things to heal my brain, and in the meantime, comforted me through prayer and the Word. While I didn't have much joy during this time, I felt His presence and was constantly aware of Him. I needed Him badly, He knew it, and He used this long trial to encourage me to depend on Him. And that I did, even though my journey towards the light felt like baby steps towards an unreachable horizon.

After four years of Lyme disease treatments, I was finally able to wean myself off of my anti-depressant, as fear and depression ceased to be my daily food.

I am so grateful that God led me out of that nightmare of a wilderness! I now know what the "real me" looks like, and am a completely different person than who I was five years ago when I was really sick. I am sane, rational, and mostly at peace. Because of what I have gone through, I know I will never take my health for granted again.

The longer I walk with God, the more I understand the amazing power of His Spirit to overcome all things, including our biochemistry. I have also learned that it takes time to understand this great power that dwells within us; to know Him and be healed—especially when the damage to our bodies and psyches has been severe. In the meantime, He will use the resources that He has provided us on earth to heal us.

I have also learned that hearing words of truth from God and acting upon them quietly chips away at the boulder of lies and depression that sit so heavily upon our hearts. We may not see the evidence of the Spirit working in our lives until we look back one, two or five years, and realize that we aren't the same people as before. It's progress, and it's hope.

Still, lifetime patterns of negativity aren't broken overnight, and the enemy is always at work to try to get us to believe lies about ourselves. So today, whenever the foul funk grips my brain, (which tends to happen less often these days, fortunately), at the first sign of negativity, I ask God to start speaking to me.

To hear from God, we must quiet our minds and shun the negative thoughts, as we focus upon Him and expect Him to speak to us. Meditation is a learned practice, and at first, we may only be able to concentrate upon Him for a few minutes or seconds, but when done daily, over time, it's possible to hear from Him and soak in His presence for extended periods of time.

When I first started asking God to speak to me, other voices in my head would compete for my attention. Over time, I learned (and am still learning!) to discern which ones are from me or the devil, and which are from God.

I have learned, for instance, that the voice of God is positive, and the voice of my thoughts, negative. So whenever I hear comforting, encouraging, wise and positive words, I know that, chances are, they are from God. Whatever words I hear that are consistent with God's Word in the Bible, I also accept as being from Him. If the voice is negative or condemning, then I know that the source is another. God's voice is never against His Word and neither is it condemning.

Bill Johnson, pastor of Bethel Church in Redding, CA, in his DVD presentation, "Recognizing His Voice" says that God's voice is always life-giving. That is, His words produce life in us, even though their initial taste may be bitter (because He is trying to impart some difficult truth to us or which doesn't initially make sense). Conversely, the enemy may feed us sweet words, but if they don't align with the Word of God or end up producing bitter fruit in our lives, then we know they aren't from God.

It's important that we examine our hearts during prayer, to make sure that our biases and wishful thinking don't get in the way of hearing from God. We must come to Him with a willingness to accept that His words won't necessarily be what we want to hear, but they will always bring light into our lives. The more we learn to surrender to Him, the freer our minds will become from biases, and the more we will accept the truth that we can hear from Him. Also, we must believe that the Creator of the universe is eager to speak to us, and that we can hear His voice just as surely as we hear the voice of our neighbor on the phone. Although God can, and occasionally does, speak in an audible voice to us, most often, His voice manifests as a quiet part of our thoughts. Distinguishing His voice from our other thoughts takes practice, but is well worth the effort.

So hearing from God is an active discipline, not a passive one, and it takes time to learn how to "tune in" to Him. Whenever I am able to do this, I hear things that are far and above more lovely, kind and optimistic than any of the knee-jerk mental garbage that fills my mind when I live unaware of my thoughts. Believing what I hear is also challenging, and I sometimes reason away God's words as a product of my wishful thinking. Yet in my wiser moments, I know that the voice that I hear during my meditative prayers is God's, because I receive wisdom, revelation, encouragement, strength and peace from it.

Following is an example of what I hear when I get quiet before God and stop letting my mind run wherever it pleases. Notice how different it is from the middle-of-the-night dialogue that I presented earlier in this section and which I sometimes get when my mind and body are sleepy and suffering.

God: "I want you to be well, but I need you to learn how to meditate upon truth. Your freedom is in knowing the truth and thinking right thoughts. In knowing the power of My Word and applying that to your life. I have great plans for you, but you must believe Me. You say you have believed me for healing, but you have only hoped for it, and countered any belief by declaring your fears that you won't be healed. Whenever you think and speak negative words, they negate your faith. Be patient, thank Me, and trust Me. Above all things, trust Me, because I will restore the years that the locusts have stolen away from you (Joel 2:25). Remember, I came to give you life, and to give it to you more abundantly! That doesn't mean a life of depression, isolation and illness. In the spiritual realm, you must believe first in order to see. Things work in reverse here. But if you choose to trust Me, I will enable you to believe. I will strengthen and uphold you with My righteous right hand, and bring knowledge of truth to your remembrance, but you must first decide to acknowledge and believe Me. You can do it. I will help you. Remember, speaking truth makes manifest things which are not yet seen. Your symptoms and circumstances aren't truth; my Word is. Speak My Word, meditate upon it, and keep it in the midst of your heart."

At times, I have struggled to accept these kinds of words. They are too beautiful; too good to be true. Besides, it has scared me to hope. In such moments, I tend to disregard what I hear and instead believe the words to be a product of my wishful thinking. At other times, I have been more receptive and willing to believe that the words that I get are from God. Then I think, "Wow, God, is this really the truth? How wonderful!" And my heart does a little dance of joy, as I allow myself to be moved by what I hear. My emotional response is mixed, based upon how much I am suffering at the time, and how willing I am to believe that He can and does speak to me. Ironically, my emotional response also depends upon the state of my biochemistry.

Whenever God's truths manage to sink into my soul, my beliefs also change, but I must continually acknowledge Him and seek Him daily if I want to remain grounded in those right beliefs, because circumstances, neurological symptoms, and the lies of the devil (who also feeds input into our minds) daily threaten to snatch them out from under me. Admittedly, my quiet life of relative solitude has made it easier for me to acknowledge God moment-by-moment and hold onto the marvelous words that I hear in the morning. But if I start skipping my prayer time, the lies creep back in, and if they meander in my mind for too long, they become full-blown creatures of destruction. Before you know it, I no longer believe God's promises. Everything and everyone around me turns a different shade of ugly, as I once again believe that God needs for me to be sick, isolated and poor, so that He might teach me a thing or two. "And nobody loves me," is the epilogue that sometimes attaches itself to this lie. What's more, my mind admonishes me to take comfort in that lie, because surely, it's for my ultimate good!

So in order to understand God's love and know His will for my life, I must challenge every despairing thought, and constantly return to the promises of peace and prosperity that He feeds me whenever I kneel silently before Him. Pursuing Him with diligence and patience is the most important thing that I can do all day.

It's frustrating when we don't hear God's voice, but it takes time to discern it, and I have found that I would give away every second of my day, just to get a word from the Creator of the universe. What could be better?

Not everyone hears complete sentences from God when they ask Him to speak. Sometimes, God reveals truth to our hearts through a Bible verse that seems to "jump off of the page" as we read it and realize that it's meant just for us. At other times, He speaks through impressions, our intuition, pictures, images, dreams and visions. He also communicates through other people, but He wants us to have a personal relationship with Him, which means that we shouldn't rely solely upon others to hear His voice. Besides, no human paints a perfect picture of God, so we need to find out for ourselves who He is, directly from Him.

He wants to show us how deeply He loves us, and that He wants to heal us. The process of knowing may take time, but He urges us to persevere, and listen with our ears, eyes and hearts wide open. He wants us to trust Him against all odds, and believe Him when He speaks, because He longs for us to hear Him.

I encourage you to kneel before Him, or just get comfortable on your bed or the floor, and spend a few minutes asking Him to speak to your heart. If you experience nothing, or your thoughts wander and/or are negative, don't give up! Keep trying. Sit for as long as you feel comfortable, and be honest with God. He can work with you wherever you are at in your walk with Him. He has no expectations of you, and only wants your willingness and desire to hear from Him. He will work out the rest, in time.

Meditating Upon His Truths

Before I surrendered my life to God, I occasionally read the Bible. Some of its words seemed condemning, bizarre, and nonsensical. Surely this book was *not* written by God, I would think, but by chauvinistic, violent white men who wanted to control humanity. In my darkened mind, full of rebelliousness and unforgiveness, I was unable to see it as God's love letter to me and I missed the true intent behind its words. And because I harbored resentment against those who had hurt me in the past, I consequently believed that if the creator of the universe was the God of the Bible, then surely, He was the greatest wounder of them all.

Only after surrendering my life to God, and accepting that I didn't know what this bizarre collection of books was about, did some of the books begin to make sense to me, and more years had to pass before I could tiptoe into the other ones. Some still contain passages that confuse me, because God hasn't yet revealed their meaning to my spirit, so I leave them for a later day. That's OK, because the Bible is an odd collection of books that can't be understood unless the Holy Spirit provides revelation of their meaning. The intent behind the words will fly high and fast over your head, if, with a humble heart, you haven't asked God for understanding. Reading the Bible with a carnal mindset just doesn't work. Also, God uses the Bible to speak to us personally. If He knows that a particular book, chapter or verse isn't relevant to our lives right now, then He won't reveal its meaning to us. Even the most brilliant theologians will admit that to read and study the Bible is to learn and accept that it will never be fully comprehended by anyone.

Yet, it's a divinely inspired collection of books in which God's person and will for humanity is revealed. When spoken and meditated upon, the Word has the ability to part seas, move mountains and alter our biochemistry, but only when the verses are relevant to our lives and their meaning is imparted to us by the Holy Spirit.

The Word makes manifest things which are not yet seen, releases good as it binds evil, and brings about God's kingdom on earth, as it destroys strongholds of darkness. The Word of God is also infused with power to dismantle the lie-based thoughts that keep us mired in disease. When we meditate upon it, the fortress that shields our hearts and minds from truth is demolished. At first, the Word may produce only tiny fissures, but with perseverance and guidance from the Spirit, the fissures become cracks, until finally, the entire fortress crumbles. Then we experience freedom, as God's light penetrates our hearts and brings our minds and bodies back to health.

So while it may seem like nothing at first, meditating upon God's Word (especially the verses regarding His promises to heal) is a powerful weapon to dismantle lie-based thinking. Provided we believe in it enough to study it on a regular basis and let it heal us.

I'm not an expert at meditating upon the Word. I get stuck in my head and the day-to-day stuff of life, and I give up when I don't experience immediate changes in my thinking. My impatience and "results-now" mindset quickly lead me to conclude that speaking God's Word is nothing more than an exercise in positive thinking, and that I'm wasting my time. Fortunately, God eventually prods me to get back on the truth wagon.

Our greatest need for truth comes whenever we start believing lies about God's plan for our lives, but we tend to turn away from the Scriptures at such times. Truth? What truth? We think. Even if we do remember the truth, the lies often come so fast and furious that they swipe it out from under us. We then stumble to pick it back up. Yet, if we have made meditating and speaking words from the Bible a habit and learn to recognize the lies for what they are, then we will have greater victory in grabbing onto verses of truth when the lies come at us.

Knowing His Love through Images, Visions, Nature and the Physical Touch of the Holy Spirit

God occasionally uses scenarios, images or scenes from my life to speak to me in prayer. These help me to know His love and will for my life. He may do the same for you, if you are open to the possibility that He can speak to you in a multitude of creative ways.

A few years ago, I embarked on a prolonged vegetable fast, with the intention of knowing God better. Fasting releases power within the spiritual realm and enables us to see and hear from Him more clearly. One day during this fast, as I was lying on my stomach in prayer, my forehead propped into my hands, God placed a vision into my mind.

The vision began with me running through a forest. Darkness enveloped me and suddenly I whacked my head on a tree trunk and fell down. I stood up, whirled around, and behind me stood Jesus, shrouded in light. He told me that I had whacked my head because I had been running too fast, away from my wounds and stuffed emotions, and He needed me to slow down so that I could be healed, once and for all— from my disease and the demons of my past.

Then a different scene flashed before me. In it, I was a little girl, and God had morphed into a tall, gentle man with sandy blond hair. He had become my earthly father and He lavished attention upon me like nobody ever had. He smoothed my hair and told me that I was beautiful. He observed me with intrigue and interest as I drew pictures with crayons. He asked me if I was hungry. If I would like to go to the park, or play with my Barbie dolls. I was in awe, as I realized that my thoughts, feelings and opinions deeply mattered to him. With a smile, he said that he delighted in me and that He loved me. He lavished attention upon me as if I were the greatest treasure in His world.

It felt odd to be treated this way. Were little girls meant to be doted upon like princesses? Then He said, "This is how I would have treated you, if I had been your earthly father."

Really? I thought, intrigued. I knew of no dad on earth who treated his child with the incredible level of love, respect and acceptance that I suddenly felt in that moment.

Then I found myself back in the forest with Jesus. We plopped down together against a tree next to a river, and He embraced me, His touch strong, yet gentle. I hugged Him back, feeling my sickness and weakness intermingling with His health and strength. Divinity met humanity. How strong He was, and how battered I was! Pain and fatigue coursed my limbs and He held me in my pain. Tears spilled from my eyes, as I realized that He knew, felt and understood the lifetime of grief that had taken up residence inside of my cells.

He said to me, "I understand why you hurt—everyone and everything that has ever hurt you is pent up inside of that body. It's not your fault that this happened to you. It's not your fault you have problems. I don't blame you for being sick. Your body and soul weren't created to endure all of this."

He didn't blame me for not being a better person and for getting sick! At that moment, I felt all of my guilt and life's regrets melting away. My chains were being broken.

Then I saw myself as a baby; a perfect, quiet, healthy creature, untouched by the world. How different I was then! Life hadn't had the opportunity to soil me yet.

With a flip of the thoughts, I then fast-forwarded thirty years, to my body of today, stressed and broken by life, and my Jesus, sad because He never wanted this to happen to me; darkened DNA, broken cells, a body, spirit and soul in dismay.

I wailed, my body wracked with sobs, and He urged me to release all of the pain that had been imprisoned there for years. As I cried, I realized that He wanted to be literally everything to me; my comforter, strength, wisdom, encouragement, healer, guide, and provider. Never had this truth touched my heart so profoundly before!

With this realization, the vision concluded but I remained in my prayer position for several minutes afterwards, absorbing the amazing reality that had just touched my heart. I wanted that feeling of God's love to stay with me forever.

In our day-to-day lives, people offer different things to us. They may give us a word of wisdom. They may provide a roof over our heads or a shoulder to cry on when we need someone to talk to. But rarely is anyone all of the things that Jesus became to me in that vision, and never do they provide them so perfectly and abundantly as He did in that brief moment for me. His love is infallible and infinite; His provision, strength, and healing are given in perfect measure. How little I had understood this in my daily life! But during that fast, I got a brief glimpse of how much God loves me and how truly, He wanted to provide for all of my needs.

Since this revelation, the enemy has challenged me in my belief that God can be my everything. So time and again, God has admonished me to go back and contemplate the vision so that I can be reminded of who He is. He has also reminded me that, although my life is far from perfect, I have come a long way since I surrendered my life to Him in 2002.

I don't know anyone who lives as the Apostle Paul, who learned to be "content with whatever I have" (Phil. 4:10-14) but this is the goal that God has in mind for His people, because true healing happens when our peace isn't shaken by life's trials. Physical healing is one of His gifts, but ultimate, body-mind-spirit healing comes from knowing how much He loves us.

I encourage you to be open to the multitude of ways in which God can speak love into your heart. He is creative and we shouldn't limit Him by assuming that the only way that He speaks to us is through circumstances or the Bible. He may want to paint pictures for you in your prayers, as He did with me. He may express His love through song lyrics that resound in your mind or in dreams that speak to your heart. When God speaks through dreams, it's often symbolically. At first, you may not recognize when your dreams are a direct message from Him, but if you practice writing them down and ask Him for revelation, or solicit help from someone skilled in dream interpretation, you may discover that this is one way in which He desires to speak to you.

Another way in which God uses images, visions and scenes from our lives to express His love to us is through Theophostic prayer. This is a type of guided prayer experience where a trained minister journeys with you into the past and asks God to reveal experiences that have created your present wounds. He or she then invites Jesus to revisit and rewrite those scenes with you, so that your wounds may be healed and beliefs reprogrammed. The TPM (Theophostic Prayer Ministry) website, defines this ministry as: "Intentional and focused prayer with the desired outcome of an authentic encounter with the presence of Christ, resulting in mind renewal and subsequent transformed life." For more information on Theophostic prayer, visit: www.theophostic.com.

God may also speak through Creation. He may take one of its elements and draw your attention to it, as a means of sending a message to you. He may, for instance, stop a sparrow before your eyes, or reveal a rainbow through your bedroom window just as a storm is raging in your heart.

Even if you miss the specific message that He is sending you through nature, the beauty of His Creation provides a powerful glimpse into His character. The mountains and roaring seas testify to His power and majesty. The sweet scent and soft colors of the rose speak of His gentleness and beauty, and the diversity of landscapes and the earth's creatures attest to His creativity. The order of nature reveals His intelligence and wisdom, and the quietness of a still forest reveals His peace.

Finally, God may speak by touching you with a physical manifestation of His Spirit in your body, mind and spirit. This often happens in Pentecostal and charismatic-type churches, but it can also happen anytime and anywhere God wants to impart a powerful revelation of His love to His children. During such manifestations, you may feel warmth or an electrical sensation in your body, accompanied by a feeling of peace or profound joy.

Sadly, most Christian churches in the United States disregard or are critical of such manifestations of the Spirit, but in most churches around the world, they are a primary way in which God expresses His love to people. In fact, according to Francis McNutt's best-selling book, *Healing,* (and as I mentioned earlier) supernatural healing and physical manifestations of the Spirit are among *the* most common ways that God introduces Himself to people in third-world nations. During my first years as a follower of Jesus, I attended churches that didn't believe in these manifestations. Over the past few years, as I have become more involved in Spirit-filled churches, my spiritual growth has skyrocketed, because I have been allowed to experience God on a deeper level.

Why? Well, who wouldn't like to experience a God hug? That's what a physical manifestation of the Spirit is sometimes like, and what I have felt in a few of my encounters with Him. The "falling down" of people that we witness televangelists performing in congregations isn't always quackery. It's God reaching out to embrace His people and fill them with a physical experience of His love, provided they are open to it.

The Vision That Enabled Me to See My Loved Ones As God Sees Them

Several years ago, a prophetic friend and spiritual mentor encouraged me to pray for my parents. So insistent was he that I do this that I became terrified that something bad would happen to them if I didn't pray. So the day I received this information, I told God that I would stay up all night if necessary, in order to receive whatever information He had regarding my parents.

At eleven p.m., I turned off my bedroom lights and sank into my bed, my back against the wall. I shut my eyes, cleared my mind and asked God to speak to me. I waited only a few minutes before scenes began appearing before my mind's eye.

In the first, my parents were holding hands and smiling, their countenances radiant. They were younger; perhaps in their early thirties. Big, bright orange and yellow butterflies fluttered about them in a turquoise sky. It seemed that they were in Heaven.

Then, my sisters and I appeared, and the five of us—my parents, along with my two sisters, Wendy and Julie, and I—grasped hands and began dancing in a circle. My sisters and I were young; maybe ages six, four and three. Then Jesus entered the circle to dance with us.

Our faces reflected a joy we had never experienced in our earthly lives. Because of this joy, we looked like entirely different people.

Then this scene morphed into another, and my parents were suddenly in God's purple-walled palace. Gold adorned His throne, and my parents stood before Him, holding hands. Their faces looked worn out by the world, but their eyes shone expectantly, like those of little children before their Daddy. I couldn't see God, but I knew He was sitting on the throne and my parents were like little figurines before Him.

Next, scenes from my childhood flashed before me, one after the other. In the first, my mother lay anxiously in bed at the hospital. She was giving birth to me, and I was arriving into the world six weeks early. My umbilical cord was choking me, and the doctors didn't know if I would survive. I glimpsed my father, wandering about the hospital, worry scrawled across his face.

A dozen subsequent scenes followed. They included: me as a baby, lying asleep against my father's chest; my father, teaching my sisters to fish; my mother, sewing me a dress and helping me to put together a poster for an art contest at school; Dad carrying me lovingly from my sister's bedroom into my own as I slept; Christmas and Dad's happy face as my sisters and I shrieked with delight over our gifts; Mom tucking me into bed at night; Dad taking us to the drive-in movie; Mom making German pancakes for breakfast; Dad teaching me arithmetic and praising me for my good grades. The images were joyous, and represented all of the wonderful things that my parents did and were for me, as well as the sacrifices that they had made for me.

Then God showed me something new; life from my parents' perspective.

He revealed their hopes and dreams for their lives as young, married adults. They had expected a prosperous life, and hoped to raise happy, successful children. They wanted to be good parents, had great aspirations for their family, and were excited about their new life together.

So they had three daughters and raised them the best that they could.

But one day, when their daughters became adults, they angrily told them about all the wrong things that they had done as parents. Bewilderment and sadness filled the hearts of the now older couple, as they wondered where they had gone wrong. Confounded, they asked themselves, "Didn't we sacrifice and work hard to provide for our kids? Didn't we all have some great times together as a family? What about all those meals we cooked, the long hours we worked to provide for them, the days we spent helping them with their homework and teaching them to swim and ride bicycles? What about the vacations to Disneyworld and Disneyland? Sure, we made mistakes, but was it really that bad? I mean, we devoted our lives to them! And what about all of the positive values that we taught them? Don't they know how much we love them?"

As I witnessed these words, I realized that God was giving me a glimpse of my parents through His eyes. He didn't see them as dysfunctional adults, but rather, as His wounded children, who had been thrown into the scary, enormous task of parenthood.

How difficult this task was! None of God's children did it superbly, and my parents had labored at it best they could, with the resources that they had had at the time. They had reared and raised three human beings in an incredibly difficult and evil world.

Then the vision changed again, and my parents were sitting on Jesus' knees; Mom on one, and Dad on the other. They were small as toddlers, but their faces were wrinkled and weary. My father wept as Jesus stroked his forehead and drew him closer to Him.

Then, in a flash, Jesus was carrying him across a beach, just like the man in the famous Footprints poem. The sun sparkled golden upon the deserted beach, and all was calm as Jesus embraced my father; his tired, worn-out child. My father dangled in his arms, but Jesus held him with great love and strength. It was as if He wasn't just carrying him, but all of his life's burdens, too.

In the next scene, Jesus stood with my mother on the beach. He drew her to Him and whispered, "You're beautiful and I love and value you for who you are."

Then it was as if God was telling me that I didn't value my parents' experiences, and I couldn't fathom all that they had suffered, but He knew and loved them infinitely, despite their mistakes.

In the next scene, I saw angels being placed around my parents' bedside; all around and on top of their house and cars. I sensed God asking me to pray protection over my parents, but not to fret over their wellbeing, because He loved them more than I, or any human being ever could, and hadn't He just shown me that they were His beloved children?

Finally, He showed me an image of Jesus on the Cross, and His final words seemed to be, "I love your parents so much that if they had been the only human beings on the planet, I would have died for them and them alone."

Then the scenes were no longer. It was twelve-thirty a.m. by the time the vision ended, and tears were streaming down my face. I had been in prayer for an hour and a half, and for the first time, I realized that I had been able to see my parents through God's eyes, instead of through my own wounded human spirit.

Another layer of bitterness lifted from my soul, as I suddenly knew that God doesn't see us as we see ourselves. His image of us is much more compassionate, kind and forgiving, and all because we are His children. Through this vision, He taught me how to have compassion upon my parents, at the same time that He showed me how great His love is towards us.

Discovering His Love Though Prophetic Words

God sometimes makes His love known to us through prophecy. More than just a means for revealing future events, God also uses prophecy to encourage us and provide us with wisdom.

Those who have learned to discern the voice of God, through experience, humility and time spent actively listening to Him, are often God's preferred instruments for relaying a message to others. Not all words that people claim to be from God are from God, however, so the veracity of any prophetic revelation should, ideally, be confirmed through a second source, such as Scripture, another person, an event, or through the fulfillment of the prophecy itself.

God has often used my spiritual mentor Rick, whose love for God runs long and deep, to help me through the hardships of illness by giving Him words of prophecy to encourage me. During my first years with Lyme disease, Rick would call me whenever I was having an exceptionally difficult day, to offer words of comfort and wisdom that

God had spoken to Him on my behalf. Rick knew when to call me because the Holy Spirit would prompt him, and I knew that I could pour out my grief, and that he wouldn't run from my pain. Always, he remained as a tree of deep roots throughout the storms of my despair. So prophecy is one of God's great tools for bringing His love and hope for healing into the human heart, but we must believe that He can speak to us through others, as well as through the Spirit that dwells within us.

I began receiving words of prophecy after I became sick with Lyme disease. I had surrendered my life to God several years prior, but it was only after I became ill that the messages started coming. The longer I walk with God, and the more I surrender to Him, the more messages I receive, and am able to discern.

All of these messages have been to encourage me, give me wisdom or help another. Most have been confirmed by a second person, which lends credibility to their validity, as sometimes, people confuse God's thoughts with their own.

About eight months ago, I received a most amazing and beautiful prophecy. During an altar call at church, as I was standing at the front of the church with about twenty other people, the pastor came over to me, and spoke the following words over me, as if they were a song. In an expressive voice, she said: "There's a song, a song of deliverance coming in the night hour, which God is going to shower upon you. There's rain coming. There's rain coming in the desert. The Lord says, 'You are hungry, and you have been thirsty. But there's a flood coming, to rain in your desert; a flood of My presence like you have never experienced before. You are My worshipper, and you have a song that has been locked up inside of you; a song of praise. And I am unlocking this song; a testimony that you will declare out to others and say, 'Come and see the salvation of your God! Because He has come to me, and as He has rained upon my life, so shall He rain upon yours!' And I will carry you away to a higher place in Me.'"

As the pastor spoke, tears filled my eyes. I knew God was speaking through her, because the words were exactly what I needed, which was to receive a profound revelation of God's presence amidst a difficult trial that I had been facing in my life at that time. I had been desperate for a deeper taste of His love, and He confirmed to me that night that it was coming! Joy filled me as I realized that He had heard the cries of my heart.

So prophecy is a powerful tool that God can use to impart His love to us, but we must be surrounded by others who believe that God can speak to us in this way if we want to receive a message through others. Some Christians believe that the Bible is the only place where God's truths are revealed. They think that He doesn't speak directly to people anymore, so if you are involved in a church whose people accept this theology, you may not receive a message from Him through others. This is because their ears may be closed off to anything that God would say to them personally.

In his DVD, "Recognizing His Voice" pastor Bill Johnson of Bethel Church in Redding, CA, says that the Bible provides principles for us to live by, but it's the voice of God (through the Holy Spirit) that gives life to these principles. Without His voice, the Scriptures can't speak to us personally and change our lives. Furthermore, we won't accurately apply their principles, and will misunderstand what God wants to say to us. Many religious wars have been caused by those who interpreted the Scriptures in the absence of revelation by the Holy Spirit.

Yet, many churches value the principles of the Bible over hearing these principles put into action by the voice of God in the present, and according to Bill Johnson, this creates religion instead of relationship with God. It also limits God's ability to speak to us personally.

Most people won't receive prophetic words unless they immerse themselves in an environment where prophecy is practiced, although God also uses people outside of the church to relay His love and concern for us, as well. If you have ever had someone come up to you and say something like, "I just have a bad feeling about this situation, be careful…" God may be using that person to communicate a message to you. But be careful about who you receive your truth from, and always verify anything that you hear from others with God yourself. He will give you an impression about whether or not the prophecy is true. Through prophecy, we can discover God's love and will for our healing, but those whom God uses to speak to us must be able to discern His voice and receive information from Him.

I encourage you to keep your eyes, heart and mind open to the possibility of receiving a message from God through other people. Don't get discouraged if He doesn't give you a word right away. He speaks to us only when we are ready and willing to hear His voice, but I believe that the more we acknowledge Him and surrender to Him, the greater the likelihood that we will receive a word from Him.

Learning About Him by "Hanging Out" With Him

On occasion, and during my worst days with Lyme disease, I used to dance with God in my living room while listening to music. I would grab a pillow and embrace it, closing my eyes as I pretended that the pillow was God. Even though my white fluffy in no way resembled the Creator of the universe, I yet believed that He was dancing with me, because I sensed His willingness and enthusiasm to embrace me and move with me under the silliest of circumstances, just because I desired to be with Him. God created humanity to be in companionship with Him, so how could He not want to dance with His children?

Once, I felt strange doing my little dance. I thought, "God has more important tasks to accomplish in the universe than pretend-dance with one of His creatures." My heart wasn't in it, but because I had been alone for days, sick and isolated in my apartment, I was desperate for a friend. Besides, another friend had urged me to "just have fun with God," because our companionship is what He most desires. What a concept! So I pushed past my strange feelings and ended up having a glorious time with Him.

But how do we be friends with God, when we live in a society that has taught us to come to Him with a sorry-please-thank you laundry list, because we think that this comprises a good relationship with our Creator? "Hanging out" with Him is a foreign concept to most of us.

I mean, what do you DO when you hang out with God? I have discovered a few activities, besides acknowledging Him in my daily tasks, but I don't do them often enough. This is sad, because they provide me with insights into His character. When I dance with the pillow, for instance, I sometimes sense His compassion enfolding me and reassuring me that He loves me and that I'm not alone.

Once, I invited Him over for dinner. I set him a place at my little coffee table in Costa Rica and acted as if He were right there with me, partaking of my meal. I went to the supermarket, and purchased wine, alfajor cookies (imported from Argentina) and all of my favorite foods. I lit candles, and I dressed up. I wanted a different experience of Him, apart from the Santa Claus that I sometimes envisioned Him as, and which I used on a daily basis to get my needs met. I wanted a God that was more than just my parachute during times of crisis—I wanted a friend.

As I ate in peaceful companionship with Him, I talked and joked with Him. I would say things like, "Hey God, are you going to eat that? Mind if I do?" as I would reach over to His plate and help myself to His chicken. (Since He wasn't literally eating the food that I had placed in front of Him)!

After dinner, I sang to Him, and envisioned Him listening to me, proud of the voice that He had given me and delighted that someone would take time out of their busy day to make Him dinner.

Sometime during the meal, though, my heart became heavy. I thought; why don't more people want to spend time with God, just to get to know Him? Why don't I want to do this? He gave us so much, and yet most of us only want His gifts, not Him. Does this make Him sad? How could it not? He is a being with feelings too, and He created us for companionship with Him. He loves to meet our needs, but also wants to be in a real relationship with us. Why, just look at Jesus. He wept. He grieved. He laughed. He rejoiced. He had compassion upon others. And if Jesus represents the most complete revelation of God's character on earth, then the emotions that He demonstrated while on earth are the emotions that God the Father and the Holy Spirit feel, too.

But some of us forget this. We think, If God is all-knowing, all-powerful and all-loving, then how is it possible for Him to crave our love, especially because it's so paltry compared to His?

Yet, the Bible says that He created us to love and glorify Him because of the love that He has for us. Deuteronomy 6:5 states, "You shall love the Lord your God with all your heart, and with all your soul, and with all your might." God wants a relationship with us, but sadly, not many people are interested in spending time with Him just for the sake of getting to know Him.

Maybe you have tried to know God personally and been frustrated with the results. You pray, but hear only a condemning voice. Or you sense nothing. He doesn't seem to be present when you call upon Him. So inviting Him over to dinner or to dance with you may seem like a foolish exercise in pretend.

Yet, He promises us that we will find Him when we seek Him with all of our heart. That implies a willingness to spend hours waiting for, and pursuing, Him. It means not giving up after a day, a week, or even months! Knowledge of His love gets revealed to us in bits n' pieces. Cultivating a relationship with Him takes time and effort, just like any other relationship, but it's funny how we will invest countless hours into our earthly relationships and so few into a relationship with God! Maybe it's because hanging out with God doesn't provide us with the same immediate gratification as our earthly relationships. He doesn't hug us like our loved ones do. He doesn't answer all of our questions when we want Him to and learning to discern His voice takes practice. His silence and invisibility confound us and our warped images of Him prevent us from seeing Him for who He truly is.

Yet, over the long haul, spending time with God can provide us with infinitely higher rewards than any earthly relationship because He is the greatest source of peace and contentment this side of Heaven. Getting to know His loving character takes time, effort and a willingness to persevere, even though He may not speak to us immediately and His presence eludes us. But we can't get to know the Creator of the universe if we only acknowledge Him in occasional bouts of hurried prayer, and especially if, during that prayer, we are the ones doing all the talking.

When I ponder the fact that God has feelings, too, and that He cares about spending time with me, it broadens my realization of His love for me. He ceases to be the distant, indifferent, yet powerful Creator who sometimes turns a deaf ear to my prayers. Instead, He becomes a close friend who wants to hear about my day, and who is eager to share with me the things that He cares about in life, too. A relationship with Him is possible and it's available to anyone who desires to know Him.

Invite Him over for dinner and believe Him to accept the invitation. You never know what amazing things He will share with you or how He will change your heart! Or stroll with Him through the park and get a glimpse of His character as He shows you the marvels of what He has created in nature. Or put on some worship music and sing to Him. You can also just sit and soak in His presence, knowing that He adores just hanging out with you. And come as you are, without pretentiousness or fear, as you would a trusted friend. Know that He's there, even if you don't feel His presence at first, because God never turns down an invitation to be with us!

Embracing the Power of Praise and Song

When struck by hardship, often the last thing we want to do is praise God. In my sicker days with Lyme, I used to say to God, "I know that I should be praising You and thanking you for my life, but...I just don't feel like telling You how great You are right now." Even though deep down, I knew that my circumstances were no reflection of His character or love towards me.

Now, whenever I have a difficult day, I recall the words of a spiritual mentor, who used to say to me, "Praise God, even if you don't feel like it, and it will change how you feel." And I find that this is sometimes true.

Praising God through song is especially powerful for lifting the heart and emotions to a higher place. Not everyone who is sick can sing—indeed, I used to have scarcely enough air in my lungs to speak, never mind sing. During such times, I would whisper, or mouth the lyrics to a song from my CD player.

The emotionalism of song is powerful, but something else happens when we praise God through our singing. We start to remember all that is good about our lives and Him, instead of focusing upon the life that we wish we had and all of the hardship of our current one. Singing, like speaking God's Word, also drives away darkness. It tears down strongholds of fear, self-pity and anger, and shoos the enemy out of our thoughts into another territory. It's a sword that beheads discouragement, despair and the lies that Satan would have us believe. Supernatural power is released when we praise God with our voices. It's a weapon as much as a tool for understanding God's great love.

Praising God can be difficult when every limb aches and the brain is in biochemical turmoil. Yet if we choose to focus on symptoms, then we will struggle to believe that He loves us and wants to heal us. I used to complain to God on a daily basis, but one day, He showed me how my venting sessions weren't helping me. I had been perusing a World Vision magazine, and as photos of starving, sick and battered children brought tears to my eyes, He reminded me that, compared to these children, circumstantially, my life had been pretty good. Up until then, I had been ungrateful towards Him because He had allowed me to suffer for so long from Lyme disease. How easy it had been to focus on what He hadn't done for me instead of what He had! How could I forget about all the countries that He had allowed me to visit during my years as a Flight Attendant? How could I not thank Him for the mind that He had given me, which enabled me to write books despite my brain fog? What about the godly people that He had put into my life to help me through the hardships of Lyme? What about the food on my plate—ever abundant—and the roof over my head? Most of us who live in developed nations take food for granted, but food is a big deal! If every person in the most impoverished nations of Africa had enough food to eat and a nice roof over their heads, they would be singing the rooftops off of their huts!

Finding reasons to be grateful towards God motivates us to praise Him when all seems dark, and changes our attitude towards Him and life. Besides, Jesus died for us and has gifted us with the privilege of spending eternity with Him in Heaven. For that reason alone, and because He is the embodiment of all that is perfect in the universe, He deserves our praise. He promises that in Heaven, there will be no more mourning and crying and pain (Revelation 21:4). In the meantime, our current suffering is just a drop in the immense bucket of joy that we will experience in the next life. Paul, in Romans 8:18, says, "I consider that the sufferings of this present time are not worth comparing with the glory about to be revealed to us."

The Bible says that God is faithful, merciful, kind, loving, compassionate, wise, powerful, patient, truthful, forgiving, and so many other wonderful things that we tend to forget about when life is hard. Most of all, He's our friend! Recalling His attributes through praise helps us to believe that He loves us and wants us to be well.

Just think: He has promised to never leave us, nor forsake us! (Hebrews 13:5). We can curse, use and ignore Him, and yet, He won't abandon us. It doesn't matter what ugly personality we don; He will forgive us for our bad hair day and welcome us back into fellowship with Him with open arms. Whatever we need, He provides in abundance, according to His will.

So we can praise Him because He loves us, no matter how many soiled thoughts fill our minds and no matter how many evil deeds we commit. We don't need to act like saints, because the gifts that He bestows upon us aren't based on our performance, but always and entirely, upon His grace. He knows our wounds. He knows we are trying. He looks upon our imperfections with compassion, not disgust or disappointment. It's impossible for Him to be disappointed in us, because Jesus' work on the Cross paid for that disappointment, a thousand times over.

We can praise Him because He created us and gave us life. While we might prefer to be with Him in Heaven, He gave us a purpose here on earth, even if we don't yet know what that purpose is. He has promised to work His will into our lives, and make us into His image, if we allow Him to.

Finally, we can praise Him for sunshine, rain, and all the "little" things. It may seem redundant and obvious to thank God for the daisy in our garden, our kind neighbor or our morning coffee, but I have been amazed at how powerful it can be to stop and consider their value. Why, most of the people in the world subsist on rice (and some don't have even that), many don't have a single friend in the world, others have lost their entire families to war and disease, and millions more are disabled and too poor to live in a warm, comfortable apartment. If we have food, shelter, and a friend or two, then truly, we are blessed!

Walking In Obedience to Him

In his book, *Experiencing Father's Embrace,* author Jack Frost describes different ways to experience God's love. Most of us hope to encounter it through a "mountaintop revelatory experience" that the Holy Spirit imparts to us, but Frost contends that we also experience His love whenever we choose to obey Him, because His love abides in us and flows through us whenever we live according to His will.

According to Frost, abiding in God's love involves three things: walking in the Spirit, having humility before God and man, and witnessing (sharing God's work in our lives) with others in a transparent manner. Following is my interpretation of what it means to do these things.

Walking in the Spirit implies acknowledging, trusting and surrendering our lives to God. It's about keeping our eyes focused upon Him, as we come to Him for wisdom and guidance in all matters. It's about a willingness to give up our time and talents for Him, loving others when it's inconvenient, and submitting all of our thoughts and activities to His lordship. This isn't easy, but as we walk in His Spirit, we learn that over the long haul, His path brings greater peace and joy than ours. Dying to the need to do life our way is the key to a prosperous life. It's also a challenging choice.

Having humility implies being able to recognize when our thoughts and actions are being soiled by impure motives, and being willing to take off the shades that protect our eyes from the light of truth. Dare we allow that light to shine into our being, and show us just how full of pride, self-righteousness, selfishness and unforgiveness we sometimes are? If we are willing, God will heal us of these unhelpful attitudes and show us that the way out of our bondage isn't found in catering to our selfishness, but rather, in rejecting it. True humility isn't about thinking less of ourselves; it's about forgetting ourselves as we get lost in God.

According to Frost, when we constantly look at other people's flaws and judge them, we aren't walking in the Spirit. We experience and reflect God's love when we develop eyes to see others as Jesus sees them. He writes in his book, "The number one hindrance to an intimate walk with God, one in which we truly know and are truly known by Him, is the absence of humility. When we are more concerned about what other people think than what God thinks of us—that is the absence of humility. When we justify our behavior, shift blame, accuse, find fault, criticize or seek to vindicate ourselves—that is the absence of humility. When we had rather be right than have relationship—that is the absence of humility. When we do not confess our sins and our failures to others—that is the absence of humility." He cites other examples of what it means to lack humility, but these are a few of the important ones.

We often blame others for our problems, or for their mistreatment of us. Being willing to scrutinize ourselves for hidden attitudes of pride, judgment and self-righteousness is key to experiencing God's power and love. If we have a tendency to think that the world is always wrong and we are always right, then we will block the flow of His love in our lives.

Finally, sharing with others the role that God has played in our lives, and especially in the development of our character, enables us to experience His love, as we recall all that He has done for us and through us. Also, when we're honest about our brokenness with others, and confess how God has healed us from our wounds and weaknesses, we testify to the power of His love to change us. And as we share our stories, that love becomes reaffirmed in us.

Being Sure of How He Wants To Bless Us

I used to tie myself up in knots over the idea of God's blessings. I would ask people, "How do you define what a blessing is? What are the "good things" that we are supposed to believe God for? How can we fully trust Him unless we know what to expect from Him?"

I would think: Christians suffer hardship, the same as those who don't acknowledge a sovereign creator. Christians get sick and depressed, too. They lose their jobs, homes and spouses, the same as everyone else. They don't get special circumstantial treatment in the game of life. Hence my frustration in trying to understand what it meant to trust God for "life abundant." What did He promise me, anyway? How could I trust Him to meet all of my needs? Being sick and isolated—was that His definition of meeting all of my needs? Was His idea of provision for me to live on the street, or in a mansion? What did it mean to be blessed? After all, blessings could imply trials and hardship, so that He might consecrate me to Him. Besides, I doubted that most people around the world who loved God and believed Him for good things lived in mansions. Fact is, most don't get enough to eat, and aren't spared the devastating effects of disease, war and other atrocities. So what did He give them, in terms of life's comforts? What could any of us who love Jesus expect from Him?

"Blessings" and "good things" are vague, even meaningless, terms for people who don't know what love looks like and who haven't experienced much of God's love. Consequently, they may not believe Him for the abundant life that He promises, because they don't know what "abundant" means, in practical terms. It might as well translate as "scarcity" to them.

After several years of trying to understand what the word "blessing" meant in God's economy, I realized that I wouldn't have asked the question in the first place if I knew how much He loved me. Since then, I have received more wisdom on the matter, in part because I have experienced His love on a deeper level.

First, and foremost, blessings are about having a prosperous soul. Prosperity of soul involves being able to experience God's presence and the character that His Spirit produces in us—the qualities of love, joy, peace, patience, kindness, goodness, faithfulness, gentleness and self-control (Galatians 5:22-23). Blessings are about abundance in the soul, mind and spirit. Because if we know how much God loves us, and if He gives us the fruit of peace and joy in knowing Him, then we can endure whatever trials life throws at us and remain relatively content. Difficult circumstances don't overwhelm us, because we believe that whatever He gives us, it will be enough. Also, circumstantial blessings become of secondary importance. Every sickness might be viewed as an opportunity to depend upon Him, and every financial or relational loss as some kind of gain for our ultimate good. Yet the things that the world calls "good" we also receive as blessings; the sleek new car, the loving wife, and the strong body. We would prefer the latter, but are content with whatever we receive, because what matters most is His presence and love, above all things.

So if people who love God all over the world starve or die of disease; if a life of blessing yet allows for immense suffering, then why believe God for anything good in the physical world? Why bother asking Him for health, a relationship, or a new car? Why not just beg for a profound love experience and be done with it?

There is no better gift than being able to remain content amidst hardship, knowing that God is taking care of us. (We may not know the precise definition of what it means to be taken care of but we are at rest, because we know that He loves us). But, fact is, God doesn't want us to suffer disease, poverty and devastation, and He desires to provide for our physical needs more than we desire to receive His gifts!

While the truth about God's provision is sometimes irreconcilable (as in the case of the starving in Sudan, North Korea and other places), in the Bible, man's obedience was often tied to what God was able to provide His people, especially in the Old Testament. Those who followed and obeyed God were protected, fed and healed. Deuteronomy Chapter 11 provides one example of this. Verses 8-9 state: "Keep then, this entire commandment that I am commanding you today, so that you may have strength to go in and occupy the land that you are crossing over to occupy, and so that you may live long in the land that the Lord swore to your ancestors to give them and to their descendents, a land flowing with milk and honey." Verse 13 states: "If you will only heed his every commandment that I am commanding you today—loving the Lord your God, and serving Him with all your heart and all your soul— then he will give the rain for your land in its season, the early rain and the later rain, and you will gather in your grain, your wine and your oil; and he will give grass in your fields for your livestock, and you will eat your fill."

God has chosen to carry out His work primarily through His people, and if we can't or won't provide for those who can't provide for themselves (as Jesus commands us to do throughout the New Testament), then His will won't be done. If we don't heal and help those who can't help themselves, then God may not be able to touch people in the places that most need His presence and provision.

Also, in the Old Testament, nations suffered due to the corruption of their leaders. The same is true today, and while it's not fair that an innocent soul who loves Jesus gets punished for the malicious acts of his or her government, God may not be able to do as much in nations where His servants aren't allowed and where leaders deny their people provision.

Yet, God is sovereign and desires to provide for our physical, spiritual, emotional and material needs, and if we cooperate with Him as a people, we will receive all that we need for an abundant, prosperous life. That means health, food, shelter and protection from the enemy of our souls. This is the second part of what it means to be "blessed" by God.

Missionary Heidi Baker, in a CBN interview entitled, "Heidi Baker: Intimacy for Miracles" says of her life in Mozambique, "If God doesn't show up, we are dead. We are dead without His presence. We need miracles to survive." But because Heidi chose to obey God and bring the gospel of Jesus Christ to this nation, the Holy Spirit now literally sustains the people there by making food multiply and by supernaturally healing them through the people on Heidi's ministry team. How much disease and starvation would be avoided if those of us who have received His Spirit provided for those who have nothing?

I have experienced financial miracles whenever I have prayed for provision, and especially throughout my trial with Lyme disease. Despite not being able to work full-time for nearly six years, I have always had a place to live, money to pay for treatments, and food on my plate. Provision comes in unexpected ways whenever I ask God for it. During my first few years with Lyme disease, I wasn't sure how I would pay for my medical treatments. More than once, I had say to God, "I have no idea how I'm going to pay my bills next week, but I'm just going to close my eyes, jump off the cliff, and trust You to catch me!"

Whenever I released my anxiety over the matter, provision came. God has used my friends and family to provide for me, but also people and organizations that don't know anything about me. For instance, I once received a large donation from AFA, the Flight Attendant union that I belonged to when I worked for United Airlines. They sent me a

$4,000 donation, which enabled me to pay my bills for several months. These kind of financial miracles have happened often over the past six years.

My trials have taught me to trust in God as my ultimate provider, because He has proven to me that He is willing to give me whatever I need to survive, and has used others to accomplish that purpose.

God's provision may mean a steady diet of white rice, especially if you don't live in North America, but as a friend once said to me, "How do you know that God can't infuse that rice with all of the nutrients that a person needs?"

He admonishes to ask, that we may receive.

Meditating upon His Love Letter

One day, while browsing the Internet, I discovered the following "love letter" from God. This letter has been reproduced from the site: http://www.FathersLoveLetter.com, and is a beautiful demonstration of God's love for humanity, based on the Scriptures. Meditating upon this letter and the Scriptures contained therein has provided me with a more upfront, close and personal look at God's love for me. Maybe it will do the same for you! But don't just read the letter; chew on the verses with your eyes closed, one by one, and ask God to speak to you personally through them.

My Child,
You may not know me,
but I know everything about you.
Psalm 139:1

I know when you sit down and when you rise up.
Psalm 139:2

I am familiar with all your ways.
Psalm 139:3

Even the very hairs on your head are numbered.

Matthew 10:29-31

For you were made in my image.
Genesis 1:27

In me you live and move and have your being.
Acts 17:28

For you are my offspring.
Acts 17:28

I knew you even before you were conceived.
Jeremiah 1:4-5

I chose you when I planned creation.
Ephesians 1:11-12

You were not a mistake,
for all your days are written in my book.
Psalm 139:15-16

I determined the exact time of your birth
and where you would live.
Acts 17:26

You are fearfully and wonderfully made.
Psalm 139:14

I knit you together in your mother's womb.
Psalm 139:13

And brought you forth on the day you were born.
Psalm 71:6

I have been misrepresented
by those who don't know me.
John 8:41-44

I am not distant and angry,
but am the complete expression of love.
1 John 4:16

And it is my desire to lavish my love on you.
1 John 3:1

Simply because you are my child
and I am your Father.
1 John 3:1

I offer you more than your earthly father ever could.
Matthew 7:11

For I am the perfect father.
Matthew 5:48

Every good gift that you receive comes from my hand.
James 1:17

For I am your provider and I meet all your needs.
Matthew 6:31-33

My plan for your future has always been filled with hope.
Jeremiah 29:11

Because I love you with an everlasting love.
Jeremiah 31:3

My thoughts toward you are countless
as the sand on the seashore.
Psalms 139:17-18

And I rejoice over you with singing.
Zephaniah 3:17

I will never stop doing good to you.
Jeremiah 32:40

For you are my treasured possession.
Exodus 19:5

I desire to establish you
with all my heart and all my soul.
Jeremiah 32:41

And I want to show you great and marvelous things.
Jeremiah 33:3

If you seek me with all your heart,
you will find me.
Deuteronomy 4:29

Delight in me and I will give you
the desires of your heart.
Psalm 37:4

For it is I who gave you those desires.
Philippians 2:13

I am able to do more for you
than you could possibly imagine.
Ephesians 3:20

For I am your greatest encourager.
2 Thessalonians 2:16-17

I am also the Father who comforts you
in all your troubles.
2 Corinthians 1:3-4

When you are brokenhearted,
I am close to you.
Psalm 34:18

As a shepherd carries a lamb,
I have carried you close to my heart.
Isaiah 40:11

One day I will wipe away
every tear from your eyes.
Revelation 21:3-4

And I'll take away all the pain
you have suffered on this earth.
Revelation 21:3-4

*I am your Father, and I love you
even as I love my son, Jesus.*
John 17:23

For in Jesus, my love for you is revealed.
John 17:26

He is the exact representation of my being.
Hebrews 1:3

*He came to demonstrate that I am for you,
not against you.*
Romans 8:31

And to tell you that I am not counting your sins.
2 Corinthians 5:18-19

Jesus died so that you and I could be reconciled.
2 Corinthians 5:18-19

*His death was the ultimate expression
of my love for you.*
1 John 4:10

*I gave up everything I loved
that I might gain your love.*
Romans 8:31-32

*If you receive the gift of my son Jesus,
you receive me.*
1 John 2:23

*And nothing will ever separate you
from my love again.*
Romans 8:38-39

*Come home and I'll throw the biggest party
heaven has ever seen.*
Luke 15:7

I have always been Father,

and will always be Father.
Ephesians 3:14-15

My question is...
Will you be my child?
John 1:12-13

I am waiting for you.
Luke 15:11-32

Love, Your Dad
Almighty God

*Father's Love Letter used by permission from Father Heart Communications, Copyright 1999-2010, www.FathersLoveLetter.com

Chapter 8

The Role of Satan and Our Biochemistry in Receiving Healing from God

How Dysfunctional Brain Biochemistry Impacts Our Relationship with God

Chronic physical illness often causes mental illness, and not just because of the devastating circumstances that disease brings into a person's life. Illness in one part of the body affects the brain (and mind), and vice versa. You can no more separate the brain (and mind) from the rest of the body than the eyeball from eyesight. They are intimately connected, and when one part of the body is afflicted by disease, then the brain and the mind are usually affected, too. The opposite is also true. As a simplified example, gut dysbiosis, (a common condition in the chronically ill that occurs when cells in the small intestine get damaged), severely affects metabolism. Nutrients aren't properly metabolized, and instead pass through the intestinal wall into the bloodstream, along with toxins, where they cause inflammation. This inflammation and intestinal dysfunction affects the brain, which then sends faulty messages to the rest of the body, causing further dysfunction in the other organs and tissues. The result is severe metabolic problems in the entire body. That is the curse of chronic disease. The effects of pathogens, toxicity and trauma in one part of the body usually cause a chain reaction in other parts, so that eventually, all systems become affected.

In chronic diseases such as Lupus, Chronic Fatigue Syndrome, Fibromyalgia, Autism, ADD, MS, Crohn's and Parkinson's, (as well as others), pathogens, inflammation, metabolic dysfunction, toxins and emotional trauma conspire to turn the brain into a biochemical disaster area, and consequently, the recipient of the dysfunction into a crazy person. And if not a crazy person, then into someone who at least thinks they are! Those of us who have suffered the effects of pathogens and toxins in the brain (such as heavy metals) are intimately acquainted with how disease can turn a sane person into a monster; how it can morph even the most peaceful of souls into near lunacy and distort the personality beyond recognition.

The negative, irrational thoughts that we experience and which are often produced by a brain that's missing what it needs to function properly can, in turn, impact our relationship with God. We may view Him in a distorted light and conclude that He doesn't love us, because our faulty biochemistry causes us to make inaccurate judgments about Him. We may feel anger, fear or depression, and blame it on a lack of faith and trust in God, when in reality, our minds just need some nutrition!

Conversely, people who have enough happiness-inducing neurotransmitters and relatively well-kept brains may believe their Spirits to be strong, when in reality, their faith is based upon emotions, rather than a solid knowledge and experience of God. And, while a prosperous relationship with God produces positive emotions, in and of themselves emotions reveal nothing about our relationship to Him.

Knowing this is helpful when symptoms cause us to despair and we chastise ourselves for not having enough faith or for not being able to rejoice and sing praises to God in our suffering. Who knows if the faith of the depressed, sick person isn't greater than that of the soul that frolics about the pulpit on Sundays, all bubbles and bounce? The opposite may be true. If we realize that the negative feelings and thoughts that we experience towards God can be due, in part, to our dysfunctional biochemistry, then we will be less inclined to accept them as true. We can say to ourselves, "I don't feel like God loves me right now, but I understand that this feeling is a product of the disease I suffer from, and is not what I truly believe. I know He loves me, even if it doesn't feel like it." This, in turn, enables us to receive from Him, because we know that what we are feeling or thinking isn't the truth about how we see Him. We also realize that He understands when our symptoms produce "lying thoughts" and He doesn't blame us for having them.

Healing the brain with natural medicine can also help us to have a sound mind and enable us to see God for who He truly is and in turn, experience a relationship with Him based on truth. In doing so, we become better equipped to receive His love and a deeper healing in our minds, spirits and bodies.

It is important to note here that God's Spirit is above the body's bio-chemistry and can control it. In those who have received a profound revelation of God's love for them, who know their identity in Christ and the power that they have been given to overcome disease by the Holy Spirit, or who have invested years in knowing and cultivating a relationship with Him, the Spirit may mitigate or overcome all mental dysfunction caused by the physical world. But the strength of our Spirits is proportionate to the degree of light and revelation that we have received from God, and the manifestation of the Spirit may be weak in those of us who are just getting to know Him or who struggle to surrender to Him. He can still overcome the schemes of the mind, but it's a battle, for sure. During my crazy years, prayer mitigated the effects of my messed-up biochemistry, but only partially compensated for it. I also needed the support of medicine to help me to cultivate a relationship with God based on truth.

In the next chapter, I offer some suggestions for healing the mind and body, outside of a supernatural encounter with God. As you heal your body's biochemistry, you may find yourself able to embrace God's love for you on a deeper level, since healing the brain, in conjunction with spiritual healing, enables the mind to produce right thoughts. Right thoughts help us to see God and the world in a more rational, loving manner, which is important for attaining intimacy with Him, and believing that He wants to heal us. Our relationship with God isn't forged out of our minds, but the Spirit cooperates with the mind, will and emotions to carry out God's works on earth. Which is why having a sound, healthy mind matters. Which is why healing is in the Atonement. You can't have prosperity of soul (the kind of healing that most Christians would agree is in the Atonement) if the biochemistry of the brain, and consequently, the mind, is such as mess that you constantly suffer from harmful, negative, angry thoughts and feelings. Jesus died so that we would be redeemed, in body, mind and spirit. In the meantime, He uses resources in nature, which He has provided for us here on earth, to help us get to the reality of the belief that He loves us; to a place where the deepest kind of healing can occur.

The Role of Satan in Our Diseases

Those who believe in the Bible as the infallible Word of God also believe that we have an adversary in this world named Satan, who dwells within the spiritual realm and whose job it is to make a mess of our lives. Since we have received God's Spirit, we can have victory over this adversary, because God's Spirit is greater than any spirit that dwells in darkness. Satan has at his command a troop of demons, which he sends out to wreak havoc in the world, and which were allowed on earth at the beginning of time because humanity chose to embrace the darkness instead of the light. The first humans, Adam and Eve, invited Satan into their lives when they chose to listen to and obey him, instead of God. In the Garden of Eden, where they lived, Satan encouraged them to eat some fruit from a tree that God had told them not to touch, but any one of us might have done the same thing.

If subjecting humanity to the wrath of Satan seems unfair, we must remember that in order for true love to exist in the world, we must have free will. We need to have the ability to choose between good and evil. God loves us so much that He wants us to love Him freely, not under compulsion, which is why He has allowed evil into the world. We chose it at the beginning of time, and we must accept the consequences of that choice now.

People sometimes become frightened at any mention of Satan, but if they only knew that he has no authority in the world except that which we grant him, then they might not be so intimidated by him. If we have accepted Jesus Christ's work on the Cross and received the Holy Spirit, we have absolute authority over Satan and his demons. In any case, he doesn't have free reign on earth, and he can't do whatever he likes to us. We can choose to reject his darkness, just as we can choose to embrace God's light.

Satan attempts to influence our thoughts and actions though, and some people blame every mishap in life and every ugly thought that they have on the influence of this nasty spirit, believing him to be the direct cause of every harmful thought, action and deed committed by humanity. Ephesians 6:12 states that, "For our struggle is not against enemies of blood and flesh, but against the rulers, against the authorities, against the cosmic powers of this present darkness, against the spiritual forces of evil in heavenly places." According to this verse, the real source of our problems is Satan, and he is, either directly or indirectly, behind every mess that humanity has ever made, but only because we have allowed him to make those messes. Every time we choose hate over love, war over peace, and selfishness over selflessness, Satan gets an invitation to wreak havoc upon our lives.

Then there are those that believe that it's unwise to look for a devil under every rock, and who acknowledge the role that other factors play in the development of harmful thought patterns and actions. I think that spiritual powers are the driving force behind all that was created and all that happens in the world, but sometimes, their influence is indirect. Taking the example of Lyme disease, rumor has it that the Lyme organism, Borrelia, was created by man to be used as a weapon of warfare, but it escaped from its biowarfare laboratory on Plum Island, Connecticut and ended up infecting thousands in the United States. (Please investigate for yourself whether this is true; I take no position either way on the issue). Supposing that this is true, we might say that the creation of the organism for use in warfare was an act of Satan but that it would escape and millions of people would become ill by it was an indirect result of his actions. Likewise, the destruction of our planet and the plethora of environmental toxins that we have created through an improper use of resources are the result of bad decisions that may have been made by minds influenced by Satan (we are all influenced by him, to varying degrees, because nobody's perfect). The diseases that have resulted from these toxins are either a direct or indirect result of the enemy's actions, since Satan can also cause disease directly (as evidenced by the book of Job in the Bible). But in our day-to-day thoughts and actions, we can choose the spiritual force that we want to agree with, and for every choice we make, there will be consequences.

So what's the role of Satan in our diseases? How do we know if our relationship with God is negatively influenced by pathogens, toxins, trauma or the devil? This is what I think may happen in many who struggle with chronic illness: the enemy of this world uses people, who, through purposeful or inadvertent actions, bring trauma and disease to our lives. As a result, we adopt destructive beliefs and thinking patterns, which lead to dysfunctional cellular processes. Satan may then capitalize on this dysfunction by affirming in our minds the veracity of the lies that we have already been programmed to believe, or by taking a biochemical imbalance and attaching a lie to the fearful or depressive emotions caused by the imbalance, so that we think, "This fear isn't the result of a biochemical imbalance, I'm just going crazy and my family is going to put me in an insane asylum!" Without God's perspective, we may then unwittingly sentence ourselves to further trauma without knowing it. So the enemy may take advantage of our biochemical imbalances by whispering lies to us, which further exacerbates our problems if we don't realize the source of the lies. In our suffering, we may hear things like: "God doesn't want you well. If He wanted you well you would have been healed by now," or, "Miracles don't happen anymore, and even if they did, surely you wouldn't receive one, because they are so few and far between."

Whenever I used to think this way, I would get discouraged and angry at God, but it was because I was listening to, and believing, the wrong voice in my head. When I finally decided to listen to, and believe, God's voice, instead of the thoughts that were produced by my feelings and the enemy's suggestions, I found myself able to refute the lies. This was difficult, since my mental symptoms affected my ability to reason and see truth, but the more I practiced refuting the lies, the more I was able to accept the truth, despite my symptoms. I would say to myself, "Okay, I know it feels like I'm going to be sick forever. I know that the enemy is taking advantage of my symptoms by suggesting that life will never get better, but I choose to believe God's truths above how I feel. These thoughts are a result of my biochemistry and the devil; they aren't the truth of what I really believe in my better days of health. So I choose to just ride out this wave of misery until it passes, because I know that God's will for me is health and that He is healing me, even though I haven't experienced the full manifestation of that healing yet."

That Satan might be allowed to capitalize on our pain would seem to add insult to injustice, but it's not God's will for us to get sucked into a vortex of tragedy, and led down the halls of Hell by the evil one. Rather, we are given knowledge of Satan and his schemes so that we might understand his role in our suffering and the power that we have to overcome his lies and attempts at coercion, because lies are his greatest weapon and the ultimate reason for all of the evil and disease that exists in the world. His number one goal is to separate us from the love of God, and he will whisper whatever lie he can come up with to get us to believe in a God that likes to see His people sick, suffering and depressed. Yet God means to give us exactly the opposite; a life of health, happiness and prosperity. We must know that He is the creator and giver of life, not death!

At other times, Satan may inflict disease directly upon people, knowing that the biochemical dysfunction which disease causes will create emotional and mental blocks to intimacy with God. But we can overcome those blocks because "...the one who is in you (us) is greater than the one who is in the world." (1 John 4:4).

We can combat the enemy's attacks by speaking words of truth or by asking God for a revelation of truth, which is an effective weapon of defense against the evil one. Praising God is likewise a powerful strategy, as the enemy can't remain in the presence of praise.

James 4:7 says that if we resist the devil, he will flee from us. Resisting his thoughts and specifically stating, "I rebuke you, Satan, in the name of Jesus," is another formidable weapon against him.

The enemy also creates what are called "strongholds in the mind." These are beliefs, patterns of thought and behavior that are more difficult to eradicate, because they have been with us for a long time and are caused, at least in part, by an evil spirit that has taken up residence in our lives. These spirits don't possess us (because no evil spirit can assume control over a person who has received the Holy Spirit), but we can be oppressed by them, since we have, figuratively speaking, "opened a door" for them to influence us. That is, we have invited them into our lives by entertaining some habitually negative attitude and/or behavior. Only through repeated prayer and fasting, and the assistance of others who are trained to "deliver" us from the influence of these spirits, can these strongholds sometimes be broken. When prayer, healing the brain with nutrition, and addressing past emotional trauma with God all fail, it may be because demonic strongholds are responsible for our inability to change our thoughts, or heal from disease.

Also, some of us are held captive by generational curses, which are handed down from one generation to the next and which manifest as some type of repeated oppression within our family line. These curses can affect multiple members of our families and wreak havoc upon our (and their) bodies, minds, or livelihoods. Anxiety, for example, is sometimes caused by a generational curse, as is alcoholism or financial ruin. We can break these curses through prayer, deliverance ministry and by refusing to participate in the sins of our family or ancestors, knowing that Jesus has freed us from these because of His work on the Cross.

A sample prayer for personal deliverance from a specific spirit might look like this:

"Heavenly Father, I repent for having entertained a spirit of _____ (say, for example, jealousy). You freed me from the power of all sin by Jesus Christ's work on the Cross, and I confess that by entertaining this sin (jealousy), I have agreed with the work of the devil, instead of your work on the Cross. From now on, I choose to reject this sin, and I curse any spirit associated with this sin, in Jesus' name. Spirit of jealousy, I command you to leave now, by the authority given to me in Christ Jesus and by the power of the Holy Spirit that resides within me. My body is the temple of the living God, and where God is, there can be no darkness. Therefore, you must go, now, in Jesus' name. Holy Spirit, fill the place in me that was occupied by this spirit, by revealing truth to my mind."

You may experience no change in your feelings after such prayers. Yet if you have prayed with a sincere heart, you can expect God to free you from the influence of whatever spirit was associated with the particular sin that you were struggling with. Once the stronghold caused by that spirit has been broken, you must feed your mind with God's truths, so that you aren't tempted to return to the faulty thinking patterns that invited the spirit into your life in the first place. So for example, in the case of jealousy, you might affirm, "The law of the Spirit of life in Christ Jesus has set me free from the law of sin and death (Romans 8:2), and I can therefore choose to reject all feelings of jealousy. Every time these feelings rise up in me, I can hand them over to God, tell Him that I don't agree with them, and He will deliver me from them. I affirm that God loves me and will provide all that I need;

therefore, I don't need to have jealous feelings towards another." You might also find verses in the Bible that mention jealousy, and recite those. For instance, Proverbs 14:30 says: "A tranquil mind gives life to the flesh, but passion (envy) makes the bones rot." Reading this verse and meditating upon the fact that envy affects physical health, for example, can provide you with further motivation to avoid it.

Sometimes, deliverance prayers need to be repeated several times, and other people may need to be involved, as there is greater power of Spirit in numbers. At the same time, we must remember that all authority on heaven and earth has been given to Jesus, and those of us who have chosen to be members of Jesus Christ's body (by surrendering our lives to God) have that same authority. The same power that raised Jesus from the dead and which can literally move mountains lives within us! The more we understand this, the more we will be able to overcome mental strongholds and the schemes of Satan.

Following is a sample prayer to break generational curses:

"Heavenly Father, I ask You to look into my past and break every agreement which was made by my ancestors and which they entered into on my behalf and which has allowed demonic spirits to afflict me and my family. Please reveal any unholy covenants or agreements to me, so that I can repent of them and cancel them, in Jesus' name, and release the affliction of the demonic upon me and my family."

For more information on the subject of deliverance, I invite you to read Francis McNutt's book *Deliverance from Evil Spirits*. This book provides a comprehensive explanation of what demonic oppression is and how to get freed from the afflictions of evil spirits. It also describes ways to discern how spiritual forces are involved in our diseases.

In Conclusion

Having right thoughts is vital for knowing the truth about who we are and how God sees us, and consequently, for being able to believe in His promises to heal us. Harmful thinking patterns result from biochemical dysfunction, unresolved emotional trauma, environmental toxins, pathogens and other disease-provoking agents, as well as from a spirit that is disconnected from God and which instead receives and accepts input from Satan. We can be healed through the natural resources that God has provided us, as well as through His Spirit, who works within us to supernaturally heal our bodies, minds and memories, and enables us to walk in the truth of His love.

Chapter 9

The Resources That God
Gave Me to Heal

Note: The medical information contained within this chapter is not in-tended to be medical advice, or to prevent, diagnose, treat and cure disease. It is only to share my opinion about certain medical treatments and is provided for informational and educational purposes only. Be sure to check with your own qualified health provider before beginning any treatment described in this chapter or before stopping or altering any diet, lifestyle or other thera-pies previously recommended to you by your health care provider. The statements in this book have not been evaluated by the FDA.

A visitation of the Holy Spirit upon our bodies, along with God's Word, persistent prayer and deliverance ministry, may be sufficient to fully heal some of us of our destructive thinking patterns and diseases. Yet most of us will also need to rely upon the resources that God has provided in the physical world—medicines, healthy food, counseling, therapies and other interventions, in order to be fully healed of our physical, spiritual and emotional ailments. I don't know why some people receive a full-on Holy Ghost healing experience, while others must use medicine and other therapies and initiatives to get well. It may be that God allows some of us to take a different path for awhile because our belief in Him as our healer is too weak, and He knows that the only way that we will respond to Him is through the resources that He has provided on earth. There are probably other reasons, which we won't fully understand this side of Heaven. In any case, He puts abundant natural resources in our paths, to heal our bodies, minds and spirits. As we make use of these resources and heal from the depression and other symptoms of chronic illness, we may find ourselves more encouraged and able to believe in His promises to fully heal us.

Following are some of the additional healing strategies that I have used over the past six years and which God has used to mend my body, spirit and mind. You may find that some of these benefit you, too.

Dietary Recommendations

First, God has taught me the value of maintaining a healthy diet. If we eat foods that come directly from the ground, our bodies can function much more effectively than if we consume foods that have been extensively processed and manipulated. I don't think that it's reasonable to expect God to heal our bodies if we fill them with processed or junk food on a daily basis. My diet today consists of fresh vegetables and fruits; organic meat, fish and chicken that is free of hormones and antibiotics; nuts and healthy grains such as brown rice, all of which contain no sugar or harmful additive chemicals; and healthy fats such as coconut and olive oil. I avoid dressings, drinks and condiments that have anything artificial added to them. When shopping for groceries, I check ingredient labels on bottles and cans, to see whether there are any chemicals or unnatural additives in the products. The more that the food has been manipulated by man, the less healthy it tends to be. Consuming natural, chemical-free foods has contributed significantly to my wellbeing.

If your dietary habits are less than optimal, consider making changes. Eating properly is one of the greatest contributors to physical and emotional wellbeing. Don't be fooled by labels which claim certain boxed and canned foods to be natural—marketers often make false claims about the contents of the products that they advertise. Don't assume that foods labeled "low-fat" and "low-calorie" (unless they are obviously natural) are healthier, either. Products with these labels tend to contain added chemicals which are poison to the body. Also, unless you are overweight, low-fat and low-calorie diets aren't necessarily good. The body needs fat, and a proper amount of healthy fat actually accelerates the metabolism! Learn to observe your body's reactions to certain foods, get educated about the contents of what's on the shelves of your supermarket, and then ask God for the discipline to change your habits. It's not easy at first, but when you see what a tremendous difference in your wellbeing that consuming the right foods makes, you may find the discipline to be well worth it.

Natural Hormones, Vitamins and Minerals

Hormonal and other nutrient deficiencies and imbalances contribute significantly to disease. Replacing these, primarily through diet, NHRT (Natural Hormone Replacement Therapy) and vitamin and herbal supplements, can facilitate healing from chronic illness. When I first became sick with Lyme disease, I learned that pathogens and trauma had caused severe nutritional deficiencies and imbalances in my body. Having a single deficiency can impact the body's processes significantly, so after numerous lab and other tests, I began to replace these nutrients and hormones. Over time, my symptoms abated.

Many of the chronically ill have HPA (hypothalamic-pituitary-adrenal) dysfunction. That is, the body's hormonal, or endocrine system, doesn't function properly. Doing thyroid and adrenal function tests, and treating for thyroid hormone and other imbalances, is particularly important. My experience has taught me that blood lab tests aren't always adequate for diagnosing adrenal and thyroid problems, and that other types of testing may be necessary. To learn more about hormone deficiencies involving the adrenals and thyroid and how to treat these, check out: *Your Thyroid and How to Keep It Healthy,* by Barry Durrant Peatfield, and *Adrenal Fatigue: The 21ˢᵗ Century Stress Syndrome,* by J. Wilson. If you are a pre-menopausal woman, *What Your Doctor May Not Tell You about Pre-Menopause,* by John R. Lee, MD, and Jess Hanley, MD, offers reliable information on how to keep your sex hormones, especially progesterone and estrogen, balanced. All of these books offer natural solutions to balancing the hormones, including bio-identical hormone replacement (in lieu of the harmful, synthetic pharmaceutical hormones that are too often prescribed to women and men). Balancing the hormones contributes powerfully to emotional and physical wellbeing.

Supplementing the body with vitamins and minerals can likewise be beneficial for restoring health. Laboratories such as SpectraCell, (www.spectracell.com) are able to measure vitamin and mineral deficiencies, as well as how well the body utilizes nutrients.

In my six years of researching medicine, I have discovered that the B-vitamins, magnesium, omega-3 fatty acids and Vitamin D, tend to be the most common nutrient deficiencies that people in westernized societies suffer from. While I wouldn't recommend taking a nutrient if you aren't sure whether you need it, certain nutrients, such as water-soluble vitamins, can be safely consumed in moderate excess, because the body will simply get rid of what it doesn't need. So if you can't afford tests, but suspect that you suffer from symptoms of a particular nutrient deficiency, you can often safely supplement for that deficiency, if it requires a water-soluble nutrient to make up for what's missing.

Fish oil is particularly helpful for healing the brain, as are B-vitamins, but all vitamins and minerals work in concert with one another, and all must be present in the body for its processes to be carried out effectively. Finding a practitioner who is competent in a kinesiology technique called "muscle testing" is another way to discern exactly what your body needs at any given time. Increasingly, medical and naturopathic doctors are learning the techniques of muscle testing, as, when perfected, these techniques tend to provide more reliable results than blood tests! It's important to find a competent practitioner though, because many people know how to muscle test, but not all do it well.

How creative God is, to show us how to discern nutrient deficiencies and disease by testing the muscle responses of our bodies to certain substances!

Herbs, Homeopathy, Pharmaceutical Medications and Energy Medicine for the Treatment of Infections

In my healing journey, I have used antibiotics, herbs and homeo-pathic remedies, as well as electromagnetic devices (note: these devices are based on physical, not spiritual energy) to eliminate the multiple infections in my body. Getting rid of the pathogens dramatically im-proved my mental, emotional and physical health, and consequently, spiritual health.

Most of the chronically ill (and the population in general) suffer from some type of pathogenic infection. The plethora of bacteria, viruses and parasites in our environment allows these things to enter and thrive in our bodies. A healthy person with a strong immune sys-tem may be able to keep such pathogens in check and prevent them from extensively harming the body, but in the chronically ill, the immune system is compromised. So whether or not your illness is the direct result of a bug, pathogenic factors may yet be contributing to your body's dysfunction.

Dormant infections become active whenever the immune system is under assault. A doctor who practices integrative medicine and who is knowledgeable about different types of remedies—natural as well as pharmaceutical—may have more to offer than the one who prefers to treat all conditions with a drug. Most doctors of integrative medicine (those who incorporate conventional, as well as natural, or "alternative" medicine into their practices) tend to look for the root cause of disease instead of just treating its symptoms. Finding doctors that practice muscle testing or who use bio-energetic devices (such as the Asyra) to test for infections is an added bonus, if not absolutely necessary for some. With these types of testing methods, doctors can go deeper and discover many infections that blood tests miss.

Strategies for Removing Environmental Toxins

Our environment is plagued with a multitude of toxins that affect the mind and body. Chemicals and heavy metals contaminate the air and our household products, as well as our food and water supply. Mold is prevalent in our homes and workplaces. Healthier people can sometimes effectively eliminate these toxins from their bodies, but the chronically ill often cannot.

In my healing journey, I have used detoxification agents such as chlorella, cilantro, glutathione, French green clay, apple pectin, minerals and anti-oxidants, to remove heavy metals and other environmental neurotoxins from my body. Saunas, ionic foot baths, coffee enemas, homeopathic drainage remedies (such as those produced by Pekana), have also assisted me in this process. A comprehensive resource on detoxification and which I highly recommend for learning more about this subject is Jacqueline Krohn and Francis Taylor's book, *Natural Detoxification.*

Numerous studies have proven that environmental contaminants, especially heavy metals, are strong contributing factors to mental illness of all kinds. Most of the chronically ill (if not most of the population) have some degree of heavy metal contamination in their bodies, and consequently, suffer from neurological symptoms. Removing metals from the body can give the immune system an immense boost in its recovery and help those who are chronically ill to recover.

Heavy metal removal is serious business, though, not to be undertaken casually or carelessly, as improper chelation protocols can redistribute metals throughout the body. For more information on how to remove these contaminants, check out Dr. Dietrich Klinghardt, MD's paper on the KPU protocol, a newly developed, but highly effective method for removing heavy metals. More information can be found at: www.neuraltherapy.com/KPUprotocol.pdf. Also, Andrew Hall Cutler, PhD, PE, has written a useful book called, *Amalgam Illness, Diagnosis and Treatment: What You Can Do to Get Better, How Your Doctor Can Help*, which provides comprehensive information on heavy metal poisoning and how to treat it.

Counseling and Books

Counseling and books on emotional healing have helped me to resolve past emotional trauma associated with my disease. If you use these as part of your healing process, make sure that you choose counselors and reading materials that have been recommended by a reputable source and which don't contradict Jesus' teachings. Look for solution-oriented resources that don't encourage you to stay stuck in your suffering and which endlessly recount the injustices that others have committed against you. Good therapists will encourage you to share your past and even enter into the experiences which caused your wounds, but with the ultimate goal of providing solutions to heal those wounds.

Some people may need to see a counselor for several months as part of their healing process, while others may require several years. There is no hard and fast rule about how long healing should take, but ultimately, the process should create positive changes in your life. As previously mentioned, the *Boundaries* book series that is written and published by Christian psychologists Drs.' Cloud and Townsend, offers Biblical solutions for healing trauma and establishing healthier relationships with others.

Other books that have helped me in my healing journey and which I highly recommend include: *Battlefield of the Mind*, by Joyce Meyer, *Healing Damaged Emotions*, by David Seamands, and *Experiencing Father's Embrace*, by Jack Frost. There are many others, but these are a few which have been very beneficial to me, along with the Bible.

Physiological Strategies that Release Trauma from the Body

Non-cognitive therapies that function on a physiological level to re-lease trauma from the cells (since memories exist in every part of the body) and reprogram the subconscious mind have sometimes been helpful for me in my healing journey. One of the more effective ones that I have used is EFT, or Emotional Freedom Technique. For more information on this simple, do-it-yourself exercise, which involves reciting positive truths as you tap different points on your body, visit: www.emofree.com. EFT can heal physical, as well as mental, symp-toms.

NET, Neuro-Emotional Technique, www.netmindbody.com is a ki-nesiology technique that can also help to release trauma from the cells. NET specifically deals with negative emotional responses to trauma which have been stored in different parts of the body. It uses muscle testing and touch to locate and release these responses, which in turn heals the body.

A Word of Warning about Energy Medicine

Some people receive healing miracles through psychics, energy medicine practitioners and intuitive healers, who harness their own energy or invoke an outside source of energy to heal their clients. While some therapies and disciplines involving the body's energy are safe (such as EFT), others are not. I believe that those that make use of the body's electrical system and its own internal energy are safe (such as acupuncture). Others involve spiritual energy, and these types of therapies can be dangerous, if you don't know where the source of the spiritual energy is coming from. This is because practitioners, in their efforts to heal by directing or channeling their energy towards pa-tients/clients, sometimes unknowingly end up harnessing spiritual powers of darkness, even when their intention is to invite positive healing energy into their practices. There is a difference between the human energy of a person and the energy of spirits which can influence and (sometimes) infect human energy, and consequently, other people. Certain energy medicine disciplines have occult origins and practitioners who use them may be inviting harmful spirits into their healing practices. The influence of these spirits is then passed on to their clients.

Just because a healer can work miracles, doesn't mean that it's good to receive healing through him or her. Evil spirits can heal the body, too, but the miracle may not last and deeper damage to the recipient's body, psyche or spirit may occur down the road, and appear months, or even years later, unbeknownst to both the healer and the person receiving healing. I speak from experience. I once received healing through a woman who was able to transfer and channel her own so-called healing energy into my body. At first, the techniques that she used to do this had a positive effect upon my healing, but I suspected that something was amiss with the process when one day, I realized that I had spent thousands of dollars just to feel moderately better. In order for the techniques to work, I also had to avoid every toxin under the sun, and if I didn't, I would "erase" the benefits of her work. You can imagine how frustrating it was to spend two hundred dollars on a healing session, only to have its effects erased by a bit of dust from the highway! But that wasn't the worst of it. During one of my sessions with this woman, I ended up developing a severe hip problem that continues to this day. I don't believe that this is the kind of treatment that God would want for His children to do—a technique that is inordinately expensive, relatively ineffective, that puts us in bondage because its success depends upon avoiding a thousand toxins, and which, in the end, causes bigger physical or spiritual problems than what we had previously! So while some physiological and energetic healing techniques are beneficial, it's important to be discerning about their origins. NET and EFT make use of the body's innate energy field; no channeling of outside energies is involved, and for that reason, I believe they are safe adjunct healing techniques.

An Exercise for Meditating Upon the Marvel of the Body

Just think; God made you to be "fearfully and wonderfully made" (Psalm 139). Consider the design of your body, how intricate and amazing its processes are and how it strenuously labors to maintain life, despite the onslaught of trauma, pathogens and environmental toxins that have come against it. The heart pumps blood throughout the body, every second from birth until death. The blood brings nutrients to the cells, and the lymphatic system carries away their waste, before the excretory organs—the kidneys, lungs, skin, liver and intestines—remove this waste from the body. The musculoskeletal system maintains the body's structure, and provides us with the ability to move. The brain orders all of the body's processes with a complexity that is beyond human comprehension.

How can we not value this marvelous work of art that God has made? Instead, when illness assails us, we often bemoan and become irritated with it, because it no longer functions properly. This is sad, because during illness, the body is running a constant marathon and deserves our congratulations for being able to function at all amidst the toxic soup that it has been fed over the years. It must work harder than the body that is free of disease, even though outward appearances would suggest that it's slothful.

In my early days with Lyme, I used to rebuke myself for lingering in bed until 10:00 AM most days. I was irritated at my body's lack of ability to perform, and I repeatedly pushed it beyond its comfort level. I often suffered an exacerbation of symptoms as a result. I would ask it to go the extra mile after it had run one hundred miles.

If my body could speak, I imagine that my heart would have cried, "Stop! Stop! I can't stand in line for this long. I don't have enough oxygen!" Or my brain might have protested, "I know you're frustrated with me because you can't remember things, but I'm doing the best I can."

What would life be like if we thanked God for the marvelous work that He has made of our bodies? Perhaps we would rest in their weaknesses, at the same time that we would know that they have a remarkable ability to be restored, through their own strength and with the help of God's Spirit. The body fights mightily for life, and is amazing in its ability to recover. Yet sometimes, the damage that we and the environment inflict upon them is overwhelming, and we need God's intervention to restore them to His beautiful, original design.

A therapist once encouraged me to talk to my body parts: to ask them how they are feeling, what they need from me, and to meditate upon their role in keeping me alive. The goal was for me to learn to have compassion upon myself and my body, because this would facilitate my healing.

The exercise seemed silly to me at first, but proved to be effective. As I practiced what the therapist taught me, unexpected emotions surfaced, as I realized how little I had appreciated what God had made of me. For instance, I noticed that I would cry whenever I meditated upon my liver. As previously mentioned, in Chinese medicine, the liver is the storehouse of rage, in addition to the organ that filters out the majority of toxins from the blood. How much my poor liver had suffered over the years! How much anger it had held and stored, so that the emotional pain wouldn't overcome me. But it paid a price for holding that anger, and its ability to filter toxins had been compromised by having to deal with emotions that should have been spent and released years ago. Add to that the abundance of toxins that it had to filter from Lyme disease, and sadness filled me at the realization of the great burden that it had borne. Borrelia neurotoxins, heavy metals, pesticides, and so many other things…and yet, I resented having to give it supplements and detoxification baths to keep it functional. In my irritation, I might as well have told it, "Why can't you just function normally, without the help of milk thistle, glutathione and castor oil packs?"

Well, that poor liver once did, but in my ingratitude, I never stopped to consider all the junk that I had fed it over the years, and how I had expected it to take the abuse as if it were superhuman. Yes, our organs are an amazing creation of God but we have dumped a world of trash upon them that they were never designed to bear.

I also cried whenever I considered the immense burden of my adrenal glands and how they had been over-stimulated by many years of living in "fight-or-flight" mode (basically, constant fear). Whenever fatigue assaulted me or my blood pressure dropped upon standing, I would think, "It's because of my weak adrenals" and quietly bemoan their inability to function properly. Doing the meditation exercise helped me to adopt a new perspective—that my adrenal glands weren't weak, but my hormonal system was never meant to bear a mind and body that were stuck in perpetual "fight or flight" mode. It could only handle so much ongoing fear, and when I added to that fear, pathogens that destroy endocrine glands, my adrenals never stood a chance at being able to do what they were designed to do.

How it must sadden God to see His perfect work destroyed by toxicity, trauma and pathogens, which have resulted from humanity's foolish decisions! We have destroyed what He intended to be perfect, but thankfully, in His mercy, He has offered us a way out by providing us with resources to reverse the damage that we have done to ourselves.

Learning to take care of and appreciate our bodies facilitates healing, as we realize how amazing God's creation is and how our bodies can overcome disease, if we are compassionate towards them. I encourage you to try the above-mentioned exercise. You may be surprised at the feelings and thoughts that come to mind. If you don't feel comfortable talking to your body, ask God to show you how marvelously He has made you, and what He would want you to know about your body that would be beneficial for your healing.

Chapter 9

How to Evaluate the Benefits of Different Healing Modalities

With all the therapies, treatments and supplements out there, it can be difficult to evaluate which ones are most beneficial. Drug and vitamin supplement companies sometimes publish and promote biased and erroneous information. Drug companies have a particularly powerful influence in the marketplace, since they can afford to spend billions of dollars to lobby lawmakers and market their products to doctors, medical schools, and ultimately, the consumer. This can lead us to make medical decisions based upon the power of their influence, rather than upon truth. Yes, drugs can be beneficial for healing, but they are not the solution to most of what ails us, as our society has been trained to believe.

When deciding upon whether a supplement or drug would be beneficial for you, it's wise to do research to find out what the alternatives are, while sifting through all the marketing hype to determine what has been most beneficial for a majority.

When trying out new therapies or treatments, research their history of success, as well as their origins. Find out how many people have received tangible benefits from them, and if anyone has been harmed as a result of practicing/using them.

Finally, is the treatment inordinately expensive? Is it excessively complicated? Does it require you to give up too much of your time? Yes, treating chronic illness can be expensive, complicated and a huge investment of time and energy, but if the treatments require you to give up other important parts of your life—your relationships and time with God, for instance, then they may not be beneficial. If the regimen is so complicated and costly that it brings you to tears, it may not be from God. If doing a therapy drains your bank account yet seems to provide only moderate benefits, then it may not be worth it. If your doctor says you need to take six dozen supplements a day (even though technically, you may need them all), you may want to rethink staying with that doctor. The body can only metabolize so many pills at once!

The aforementioned are just a few factors to consider when determining whether a particular healing strategy would benefit you. You may want to ask God about others to consider before embarking upon a treatment plan.

Chapter 10

To Take Medicine or Not Take Medicine

Proponents of faith healing sometimes contend that taking medicine negates our ability to have faith in God for a miracle. They argue that when we take medicine or do treatments, our hope becomes focused upon those treatments instead of upon God. I agree that it's tempting to place our hope in whatever strategy we use to better our health. We take drugs and can't help but wonder about their effects upon our bodies; we spend time thinking about what we should be doing differently to relieve our symptoms, and we invest endless hours into doing treatments and going to doctors. Our thoughts naturally become centered upon our illnesses and remedies. We may dialogue with others about our treatments when they ask us how we feel, or we may spend hours researching the next latest, greatest treatment. So every minute that we devote to thoughts of disease and treatments is one less minute that we have to think about God and His ability to heal us supernaturally. It's just the way it is.

We may argue that God is blessing our treatments and insist that our ultimate hope is in Him, and while this may be true, if our thoughts are more about our symptoms and treatments, then we might not be placing our hope in Him as much as we think. If we constantly wonder whether or not we are doing the right thing, are always desperately searching for the next drug or stressing over the results of our remedies, our hope might not be in God as much as in the treatments. Making medical decisions can be agonizing and difficult, but if our life's hours are spent in constant striving over them, then this is a problem. Therefore, it can be difficult to believe God for a miracle and place our hope for healing in Him if we do medical treatments, especially if those treatments require a huge investment of our time, thought and energy.

On the other hand, it may be unwise to not take medicine, in order to place our hope more fully in God. If we have a life-threatening medical condition or one that causes the body to quickly degenerate, stopping treatments could jeopardize our life, especially since God's healing timetable is almost always different than ours. Unbeknownst to us, He may be waiting for us to release unforgiveness against our neighbor or have some other purpose to accomplish through our illness before we can be healed. So, stopping medical treatments may be a presumptuous move on our part. Also, God does use medicine to fully heal some people, and we must be open to the possibility that this could be His chosen method for healing us (provided we understand that the blessing of the treatment to our bodies is ultimately up to Him).

In the end, taking medicine is a personal decision. Some people have stopped doing treatments because they were fully convinced that God would heal them right away. And sometimes, He has. Other people have felt led to continue medical treatments, and this has been for them, the best decision that they could possibly make.

Another question remains, though. If we do treatments at the same time that we decide to hope in God for a miracle, how do we keep our hope focused upon Him, and not the treatments?

If you suffer from an illness that requires a lot of maintenance or ongoing treatment, this can be incredibly difficult. I have found that resisting the urge to discuss my treatment protocol and complain about or discuss my symptoms with others has been a powerful first step to steering my mind away from thoughts of treatment and disease. It's not easy to do this if your illness and treatments have become the focus of your life. It requires a concerted effort to be mindful of your thoughts and conversations with others. If you think you have nothing else to talk about because life has afforded you little opportunity to do much besides treat your disease, try asking others about their lives. Spend time with friends and family who don't suffer from the same disease as you, because inevitably, spending time with other sick people (granted, there is a time and place for this) creates an open door for you to focus upon your symptoms. As mentioned in preceding chapters, spending more time with God and reading books that have nothing to do with disease and which instead build up faith for healing are beneficial, as is resisting the temptation to worry and fret over the effects of the remedies that you're taking.

When you do treatments, pray and gaze into the face of God. Say something to Him that will steer your brain away from the temptation to analyze your treatments. Once you understand what your symptoms are and where they are coming from, try to focus on something else when they come up. Let them inform you as to what you need to do treatment-wise, but don't let them overpower your world, when focusing on them won't serve you. They may scream to be heard 24-7, but every time pain stabs you in the chest; every time your stomach hurts or your ears ring, thank God for your healing. Recite one of God's truths about healing and meditate upon what it means personally for you.

All of these strategies require mindfulness, which is only possible when we focus upon God and ask Him to guide our thoughts, as He gives us words to replace our habitual songs of self-analysis.

Finally, it may be appropriate to stop medical treatments, if the treatments aren't working, are causing more damage to your body and spirit, or are interfering with your ability to rely on God for healing. If your medical treatments are helping you, I personally believe that it would be unwise to stop them. Instead, learn how to practice the above-mentioned strategies for putting your faith in God, while continuing under your doctor's care.

Chapter 11

Believing God for a Miracle

Some ministers who have been used by God to heal multitudes argue that if we want to receive a miracle from God, then we must be certain that healing was a guaranteed gift given to us by Christ's work on the Cross. They contend that any doubts concerning His will in the matter will block us from receiving a miracle.

But what if you have believed and not received a miracle? Maybe you've attended many healing services and not been made well. Or you know people who believed God for a miracle and still died. Or you are just too afraid to hope, because shoot—doesn't it hurt when the miracle is always for someone else?

How do we reconcile the paradox of God's promises with the fact that some people don't get healed supernaturally or by medicine, even when their faith is sky high? How do we reconcile belief in God's promises to heal us with the possibility that He may have reasons for allowing our healing to be delayed?

This is what I believe. Attaining anything worthwhile in life involves risk. Usually, the greater the risk we take, the greater the potential reward. Personally, I have decided to risk believing God for a healing miracle. This has meant putting my expectations of God on the line, and risking the possibility of my heart getting smashed to pieces if He doesn't come through for me in the way that I would like. But I think that the risk is worth it, because even though not all of us will be healed supernaturally, I believe that God wants for all of us to be well—in body, mind and spirit. And I believe that He will do whatever it takes to help us achieve full health.

If I don't receive my miracle, I will be disappointed, but I won't flagellate myself for not having enough faith. Because I now know that receiving God's healing isn't just about having enough faith. If I keep that thought at the back of my mind, perhaps it will serve as a cushion for my faith, if my hopes for a miracle get dashed down the road. If I'm not fully healed, I won't blame myself and assume that I did something wrong, since, and as a good friend in Atlanta who has attended multitudes of healing services once said to me, "I've seen some of the holiest people die in their diseases, and some of the ungodliest of souls receive miracles."

But I tuck this thought away for a rainy day, because it doesn't serve me today. Today I need to have faith for a miracle, which requires me to focus my eyes upon a loving God who is willing and able to heal people supernaturally—and with medicine. I may ask Him to reveal whether something in my life is blocking my healing, but I keep my gaze fixed squarely upon Him, not my inadequacies. Because it is my faith in His love and promises, not faith in my faith, that produces the faith that I need for healing!

As I anxiously await that miracle, I praise Him with a joyful heart. Because I believe that He wants to heal me fully, in body, soul and spirit. I have already experienced several miracles in my body and spirit during the process of writing this book, and I believe that it's just a matter of time before I will be fully restored to health. In my heart, I believe that He has given me the gift of healing through His work on the Cross, and I just need to keep my attention fixed on His love and promises as I await the complete manifestation of that healing.

I think that this is a healthy way to have faith in God for a miracle. It's less likely to produce disappointment and self-doubt than if we believe that we must be healed, always, forever, and right now. Because if we adopt that philosophy, then we will conclude that we have a serious faith problem or that God really doesn't want us to be well. Sometimes, doubts do block us from receiving, and God may need for us to forgive someone or focus less upon our symptoms—but if we ask Him to remove our mental roadblocks, He is faithful and will guide us to wherever we need to go. His Spirit works within us to do all things, including developing the ability to receive His love and healing.

At the same time that we believe God for healing, we must recognize that He is sovereign, and that His thoughts are not our thoughts, neither are His ways ours, and there is sometimes no rhyme or reason to how or why or when He chooses to heal us. We want a God that fits within the box of our expectations, but if we could keep Him within the confines of our cardboard squares, then we would have no need for faith. If receiving a miracle from Him boiled down to a mastering a predictable formula that worked every time, then we would seek to know the formula, not Him.

Not everyone who loves God is healed in their physical bodies, and sometimes, there is no apparent explanation why. The fact is, God colors outside the lines, at the same time that He gives us promises that fit beautifully within the confines of our faith.

If you don't have faith in God's love and desire to heal you, ask Him to impart it to you. Ask Him to show you the path that you are meant to pursue, and then begin walking it. Take a risk, knowing that He will do the absolute best thing for you. And know that He loves you the same, miracle or no miracle. Besides, the real miracle isn't your physical healing—it's experiencing His love. And while He died on the Cross so that we might enjoy Heaven on Earth, the fullness of His love will only be revealed to us in its entirety in the Afterlife; a place where there will be no more remembrances of pain and disease, and where we will have the privilege of rolling in the full revelation of His love and health, forever.

Appendix

The Healing Testimony of Terry Wilson

*Note: Terry's last name has been changed to protect his identity

Recently, I had the privilege of interviewing a man who has been used powerfully by God throughout his life to heal multitudes. His name is Terry, and he's a good friend of my spiritual mentor, Rick. As many powerfully anointed ministers, however, Terry suffered great hardships for many years before God led him into his privileged role as a healer.

The trials started at his birth. Terry entered into the world as a "blue baby." His blood couldn't effectively deliver oxygen to his tissues, so he was given a blood transfusion, which caused him to suffer from toxic shock syndrome. Shortly thereafter, he came down with double pneumonia. As a result of these trials, his kidneys and liver nearly shut down. He also became severely anemic and suffered from neuralgia (nerve damage). Within the first year of his life, Terry almost died, three times. Yet these bouts with infirmity were only the beginning of his troubles.

Scarlet fever, rheumatic fever, scarlatina, bronchial asthma and double pneumonia marked Terry's early childhood years. Some of these infections caused fever burns to his brain, and they also caused him to develop a hole in his heart. He also suffered a bout with polio, but God healed him from this and all of the other maladies—supernaturally and through medicine.

Terry was ten years old before he realized that there was life outside of a hospital room. Yet his health battles continued. Around the age of ten, he developed astigmatism in his eyes, which God miraculously healed.

As an adolescent, he found himself stumbling into accident after accident. In one, he ended up injuring himself in the throat with a spear that he had made out of a broomstick. He ripped his larynx, which caused him to hemorrhage and created blood clots in his mouth and throat. Fortunately, he healed from this accident without too many problems. In another accident, and at the age of fifteen, he fell through a window and ended up slicing four inches of flesh off of his forearm! In an accident previous to the one in which he catapulted out the window, his arm got stuck in a washing machine roller (the kind that were used 40-50 years ago), which had the effect of stretching the skin from his forearm up into his bicep. So after the window accident, doctors were able to take the "extra" skin that had accumulated on his bicep from the washing machine accident, and graft it onto the lower part of his arm, but unfortunately, it was only skin. He had no nerves, muscles, ligaments or tendons in his arm.

Terry cried out to God to heal him. He knew of his God's great power and willingness to heal, since He had healed him of a multitude of sicknesses earlier in life. So shortly after this, he went to the doctor, and the doctor prayed for him. As he did, to his astonishment, Terry began to experience extreme pain in his hands, which he likened to "skewers with hot coals being shoved into his fingers."! What he didn't realize was that God was performing a healing miracle in his arm and was re-growing all of the muscles, nerves, ligaments and tendons.

Following the prayer, the doctor examined Terry's arm, then began to do a little dance in his office, along with one of his assistants. Terry, confounded, asked the doctor what was going on—after all, he had just experienced one of the worst pains of his life! The doctor, smiling, informed him that God had just healed his arm and re-grown all of the nerves, ligaments, tendons and muscles. Terry wondered how this was possible, since he still wasn't able to move his arm, but the doctor explained that he would need to re-train his mind to use the arm again. And so it was, after a period of time, that Terry regained the use of his arm, thanks to God's creative miracle.

But God intended to show His amazing power and love towards Terry in even greater ways. His astonishing works in Terry's life were only beginning.

As a teenager, Terry always had to wear his brothers' tattered hand-me-down clothes. Wearing worn-out clothes bothered him, so one day he asked God if He would do something about that. God's creative response wasn't just to provide Terry with a new wardrobe—but to grant him a major growth spurt one summer, in which he grew four inches! After this growth spurt, Terry stood taller than all of his brothers, and his parents were obliged to provide him with new clothes.

As a result of this growth spurt, Terry believes that he also acquired an extra set of ribs! Unfortunately, down the road, as a young adult, this caused him problems when he became a bodybuilder. He built up his arms so much that they began to constrict the arteries in his right arm and block the flow of blood into that arm. As he lost use of his right arm, once again, he asked God to heal him, and once again—God did.

But the battles with his arm weren't over. In 1967, at the age of twenty, Terry joined the army and underwent military training to go to Vietnam. During his training, he pulled some tendons in the arm. He asked God to heal him, but this time, God healed him only partially, and as a result, Terry was given a medical discharge from the army. He claims that the partial healing happened because God wanted to show him that he didn't want him just "taking off and doing whatever he wanted, whenever he felt like it." In other words, God wanted him to surrender to Him and stop living his life independently of Him. Sure,

Terry believed in God and recognized His healing power, but he still didn't have a strong personal relationship with his creator.

Shortly after leaving the army, Terry married a childhood friend and they had two children. God blessed him richly, and at this point in his life, everything that he put his hand to seemed to prosper. The blessings began with his new family, but extended into his work life, where God performed miracles just as amazing as those that he had experienced in his physical body growing up.

At the age of twenty-five, Terry was hired as an engineer for an aeronautical space firm. This in itself was a miracle, because he had never been to college. Not only that, but he passed the company's engineering test with a perfect score. Thousands of engineers at the firm had taken the same test as Terry, but only five had ever received a perfect score. Terry, having never gone to college, was one of them. It was only because of God's divine favor that he was able to pass this test and work in such a privileged position, among Master's and PhD graduates.

During his eight years as an engineer, Terry worked on a number of important programs, including the Space Shuttle, Stealth Bomber, and AWACS (airborne warning and control system) surveillance. He used the money that he earned from this job to repay his father for all of the medical bills that he had accumulated throughout his life!

Unfortunately, the enemy wasn't done trying to wreak havoc upon Terry's health. While God had blessed him abundantly in his personal and work life, around the time that he began working for the aeronautical space firm, he also developed a brain tumor. He decided not to tell his family about it because, as he claims, he didn't want them to pity him. Sadly, he believed that God was now killing him because of his sin. Yes, God had healed him of many maladies throughout his life, but he still didn't fully understand the grace that had been given to him because of Jesus' work on the Cross. He didn't know that God doesn't punish people with disease for their mistakes!

Fortunately, his growing brain tumor didn't impede his ability to work, and his mind remained sound. Having had so many attacks upon his brain throughout his life (i.e., fever burns at birth), Terry believes that it was only by the grace of God that his mind always functioned well.

But the tumor affected his life in other ways, and one day, during a fight with his wife, he blacked out.

When he regained consciousness, he found himself lying at the bottom of the staircase in his house. He looked around, but his wife was nowhere in sight. Alarmed, he noticed that all of the cabinet doors in the kitchen had been torn off, and that fragments of broken dishes were scattered about everywhere. Bloody handprints spotted the walls, cabinets and doors. There were holes in the walls, and all of the doors had been ripped off of their hinges.

At first, Terry believed that someone had knocked him out and attacked his family. Terrified, he called his mom and asked her what had happened. The anxious reply was, "Your wife and kids are in the hospital. You beat them within nearly an inch of their lives!"

Terry couldn't believe his ears. Reeling from devastation, he went back into the house and found his revolver. He put six shells into its chamber and was about to put the gun to his head, when a voice, clear as day, came to him in his thoughts and said, "You can't do this. You can't go out this way. This isn't an honorable way to die. You have to make peace with your brother first." Terry had been estranged from his brother for a long time, so the words made sense to him. He didn't know, however, that the voice that had spoken to him was God.

But it convinced him, and he picked up the phone to call his brother, who, incidentally, knew God's voice well. And God had told him to stay home that night to receive Terry's phone call, though he didn't know why Terry meant to call him. Terry told his brother about what had happened, and his brother called two ministers to come down to Terry's house to pray for him.

Terry met with the ministers, who prayed over him with compassion. They began the prayer by saying, "Our Father..." and at those first words, Terry felt a 300-pound weight being lifted off of his shoulders, at the same time that he felt the brain tumor shrinking in his head! Thoughts of suicide left him, and with a heart of contrition, he repented for what he had done to his family, as with deep gratitude, he thanked God for sparing his life.

Miraculously, God also healed Terry's wife and children. Yet perhaps the even greater miracle was that his wife decided to forgive him after he had nearly beaten her and their two children to death! Not only did she forgive him, but God enabled her to trust him again, and they ended up having a third child together.

The enemy had plans to destroy Terry and his family, but God took the situation and completely redeemed it, in a way that defies human comprehension. Only a God of miracles could heal a brain tumor. Only a God of miracles could completely heal an entire family that had been beaten to death by their husband and father! Only a God of miracles could enable that family to love and trust him again.

Following this horrific event, Terry began to attend church, but he still didn't understand what it meant to have a personal relationship with God, and to accept Jesus as the Lord and Savior of his life. Consequently, he didn't have the Holy Spirit abiding within him, either (since receiving the Holy Spirit results from accepting Jesus' sacrifice and making Him Lord over one's life). What he hadn't known when he attacked his family, was that he had been possessed by a demon, and that he still carried this, and other, demons with him. It wasn't Terry that had attacked his family; it was a spirit of darkness that had overcome him.

So despite the fact that he attended church and had every intention of living an upright life, the demons were allowed to continue wreaking havoc upon his life, and he ended up having an affair on his wife. He began to feel, as he describes it, "like a piece of driftwood," with no purpose in life.

So one day, at the age of thirty, and still married to his wife, he had a discussion with a close friend about God on the subject of why we (humans) are made and what our purpose is on this earth. He had been walking with his friend in the mountains, and their discussion culminated in Terry crying out for God on a mountaintop, because he was desperate for some kind of knowledge that he hadn't ever received before. He was tired of feeling like a piece of driftwood, and he said, "God, I prayed for all of these healings and they happened…but what is my purpose in life? Please show me!"

Well, God heard his prayer and he showed Terry that He wasn't angry at him for all of the mistakes that he had made in life; far from it! Instead, he realized Terry's desperate need for redemption, and in response to his plea, the Holy Spirit touched him powerfully in that moment, and delivered him from all of his demons and wounds, physical as well as emotional, in a way that he had never been delivered before. He was now free, completely.

From that day on, he began to experience the world and life through a new set of eyes and a new set of ears, as the Holy Spirit came to live inside of him. Along with these new eyes and ears came the ability to literally see angels and demons around and upon people, which was a gift that God had given him so that he might deliver others from their demons.

After his experience on the mountaintop, Terry's life began to change again. At first, he began to have more Job-like experiences. (The book of Job in the Bible explains how one of the world's most righteous men was afflicted terribly by Satan, but how God restored to him double all that he had lost in life as a result of the enemy's schemes). First, all of the appliances in his house broke! Was it a coincidence, or were the powers of darkness not happy about his newfound freedom and the multitude of ways in which God would now use him to help others? The next thing that happened was that his wife divorced him, and two of his children became terminally ill; one with a muscle disease, and the other, with an incurable blood disease.

But the God of miracles kept showing up, faithfully and in great power, to redeem Terry and his family from the endless assaults and attacks of the enemy upon his and their lives. And once again, God supernaturally healed his children.

Subsequently, God began to use him to heal people from their physical, emotional and spiritual wounds. Terry allowed God to use him as a healer, but told Him that he didn't want Him to put him in the spotlight, because he didn't want the glory for any of the amazing healings that God was starting to perform through him.

As part of his healing ministry, God used him to deliver people of demonic oppression. Terry would call things into existence which were not yet in existence (healings, for example), through God's word, since God promised that His followers would be able to do this by the Holy Spirit. (Romans 4:17).

And over the next thirty years, God used him to heal multitudes. Not ten, twenty, or even twelve hundred people...but multitudes. His ministry included working as a chaplain for the Department of Corrections, as well as for hospitals, prisons and nursing homes. He also worked in a boys' home; a refuge for troubled and abused kids, where God used him to heal those who stayed there of their emotional and physical wounds. At one stage during his career, he ended up as the director of a child placement agency, where he helped to find homes for foster kids.

During his thirty years as a chaplain, Terry didn't receive a single paycheck for his work. Yet God always provided for his needs through donations and charity.

Some of the healings which God has used him for over the years are truly astounding—nothing that could be accomplished through human effort or energy. For example, one man whom he prayed for had a damaged heart, a missing arm and teeth, and problems with his eyes. And God healed every single one of his infirmities through Terry! Terry claims that he had faith for God to re-grow the man's arm because of his experience of having his own arm miraculously restored.

On another occasion, God used Terry to heal a wheelchair-bound woman with whom he had worked at the child placement agency. One night, after a company Christmas party, Terry prayed over her, and afterwards, the woman rose from her wheelchair. So amazing was this miracle that, after Terry witnessed it, he dashed down the street, ecstatic and overjoyed at what God had done for his friend.

So how many people has God used Terry to heal? Thousands. He doesn't know exactly how many, but the numbers are high. When I asked him how he has managed to stay out of the spotlight with a record like that, he replied that God had agreed to keep his ministry a secret, because he had told Him that he didn't want to receive any glory for the healings that He was doing through him. He didn't want to become proud and take the credit for God's work. Because in reality, Terry wasn't the healer; God was.

Terry believes that God sometimes delays our healing to teach others around us something. For instance, He may allow us to suffer for awhile so that we may learn to give consolation to other people who are sick and suffering. There may be other purposes through our trials of illness, as well.

May Terry's journey be an inspiration to those of you who are struggling to regain your health! His story is a perfect example of how God can take our battles with disease and use them for good, and how He is willing to miraculously heal—over and over again.

Terry's life is also a reflection of the profound truth that sometimes, the greater the battles we face in life, the greater the purpose and redemptive plan that God has for our lives. Also, His gifts are given to us by His grace, not by our works. Terry suffered incredible hardships in his life, but was rewarded with one of the greatest honors that can be bestowed upon man—the privilege of healing thousands of people through God's power, and sharing with them His redemptive plan for humanity. God's work in Terry also proves how completely God can redeem a life that has been broken by disease and devastation.

Ultimately, Terry believes that healing is part of the gift that God gave us through Jesus' work on the Cross, but we must sometimes contend for that gift. Because Jesus promised those who would believe in Him and receive the Holy Spirit that, "… they (His followers) shall take up serpents, and if they drink any deadly thing, it shall in no wise hurt them; they shall lay hands on the sick, and they shall recover." (Mark 16:18).

Bibliography

Adams, Berry. "The Father's Love Letter," copyright © 1999, Father Heart Communications, www.FathersLoveLetter.com. Used by permission.

Baker, Heidi and Rolland. *Expecting Miracles.* (Grand Rapids, Michigan: Chosen Books, 2007).

Bosworth, F.F. *Christ the Healer.* (Grand Rapids, Michigan: Chosen Books, 2008).

Clark, Randy. *There Is More.* (Mechanicsburg, Pennsylvania: Global Awakening, 2006).

Cloud, Henry and John Townsend. *Boundaries: When to Say Yes, When to Say No-To Take Control of Your Life.* (Grand Rapids, Michigan: Zondervan, 1992).

Cloud, Henry and John Townsend. *Safe People: How to Find Relationships That Are Good for You and Avoid Those That Aren't.* (Grand Rapids, Michigan: Zondervan, 1996).

Frost, Jack. *Experiencing Father's Embrace.* (Shippensburg, Pennsylvania: Destiny Image Publishers, Inc., 1977).

Hunter, Joan. *Power To Heal.* (New Kensington, Pennsylvania: Whitaker House, 2009).

Johnson, Bill. *The Supernatural Power of A Transformed Mind.* (Shippensburg, Pennsylvania: Destiny Image Publishers, Inc., 2005).

Johnson, Bill. *When Heaven Invades Earth.* (Shippensburg, Pennsylvania: Destiny Image Publishers, Inc., 2003).

Meyer, Joyce. *Battlefield of the Mind.* (New York, New York: Warner Books, Inc., 1995).

McNutt, Francis. *Healing.* (Notre Dame, Indiana: Ave Maria Press, 1999).

Murray, Andrew. *Divine Healing.* (United Kingdom: Diggory Press, 2007).

Nee, Watchman. *The Spiritual Man.* (Richmond, Virginia: Christian Fellowship Publishers, 1968).

Nee, Watchman. *The Normal Christian Life.* (Richmond, Virginia: Christian Fellowship Publishers, 1968).

Prince, Joseph. *Destined to Reign.* (Tulsa, Oklahoma: Harrison House, 2008).

Sapp, Roger. *Beyond a Shadow of A Doubt.* (Southlake, Texas: All Nations Publications, 2001).

Seamands, David A. *Healing for Damaged Emotions.* (Colorado Springs, Colorado: Chariot Victor Publishing, 1991).

Stone, Perry. *The Meal That Heals: Enjoying Intimate, Daily Communion with God.* (Lake Mary, Florida: Charisma House, 2008).

Wigglesworth, Smith. *Smith Wigglesworth on Healing.* (New Kensington, Pennsylvania: Whitaker House, 1999).

Wigglesworth, Smith. *Ever Increasing Faith.* (New Kensington, Pennsylvania: Whitaker House, 2001).

Wright, Henry. *A More Excellent Way.* (Thomaston, Georgia: Pleasant Valley Publications, 2003).

Venter, Alexander. *Doing Healing.* (Cape Town, South Africa: Vineyard International Publishing, 2009).

Johnson, Bill. Healing: Our Neglected Birthright. CD. Bill Johnson Ministries, Redding, CA.

Johnson, Bill. Recognizing His Voice. DVD. Bill Johnson Ministries, Redding, CA.

Wommack, Andrew. God Wants You Well. Andrew Wommack Ministries, Inc. Copyright © 2002. Colorado Springs, Colorado.

Clark, Randy and Bill Johnson. "School of Healing and Impartation." Global Awakening. Resurrection Fellowship, Loveland, CO. 10-13 Mar. 2010

Hunter, Joan. "Heaven Invasion." Joan Hunter Ministries. Power Invasion Ministries, Denver, CO. 22-25 Jan. 2010

About the Author

Connie Strasheim was born in 1974 and raised in Denver, Colorado, but spent nearly a decade of her thirty-six years living in other places, including New York, New Jersey, Costa Rica, Argentina and the United Kingdom.

In September, 2004, Connie became disabled by chronic Lyme disease and had to quit her job as a flight attendant for United Airlines. She became a full-time medical researcher and devoted the following six years of her life to fervently pursuing healing, through medicine and her relationship with God, while working on a limited basis as a medical interpreter and private Spanish instructor.

Her research finally led her to publish two books on Lyme disease, including *Insights Into Lyme Disease Treatment: Thirteen Lyme-Literate Health Care Practitioners Share Their Healing Strategies,* and *The Lyme Disease Survival Guide: Physical, Lifestyle and Emotional Strategies for Healing.* She is currently writing a book on cancer, as she continues her research into healing.

Connie ministers to the sick on a regular basis, and conducts a bi-monthly conference call prayer group to pray for the chronically ill around the United States. She also leads a healing group at her local church in Denver. Prior to becoming chronically ill with Lyme disease in 2004, she participated in and led missions trips to Ecuador, Colombia, Guatemala, El Salvador and Bolivia. She has traveled to over fifty countries and has developed a passion for serving the suffering in underdeveloped nations. She ultimately hopes to continue to bring God's love and healing to these people, even as she serves those in her own community.

You can purchase Connie's Lyme disease books and read her Lyme-related blog at www.LymeBytes.blogspot.com.

CPSIA information can be obtained at www.ICGtesting.com
Printed in the USA
BVOW031458260613

324351BV00003B/767/P